RAPID

ACLS

T0130959

Revised Second Edition

Barbara Aehlert, RN, BSPA

Southwest EMS Education, Inc.
Phoenix, Arizona/Pursley, Texas

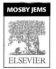

MOSBY JEMS

ELSEVIER

MOSBY JEMS
ELSEVIER

11830 Westline Industrial Drive
St. Louis, Missouri 63146

RAPID ACLS   ISBN-13: 978-0-323-08320-1
Revised Second Edition

Notice

Knowledge and best practice in this field are constantly
changing. As new research and experience broaden our
knowledge, changes in practice, treatment and drug therapy
may become necessary or appropriate. Readers are advised to
check the most current information provided (i) on procedures
featured or (ii) by the manufacturer of each product to be
administered, to verify the recommended dose or formula, the
method and duration of administration, and contraindications.
It is the responsibility of the practitioners, relying on their own
experience and knowledge of the patient, to make diagnoses,
to determine dosages and the best treatment for each
individual patient, and to take all appropriate safety
precautions. To the fullest extent of the law, neither the
Publisher nor the Author assumes any liability for any injury
and/or damage to persons or property arising out or related to
any use of the material contained in this book.

Publisher and Vice President: Andrew Allen
Managing Editor: Laura Bayless
Associate Developmental Editor: Mary Jo adams
Project Manager: Stephen Bancroft
Cover Designer: MWdesign, Inc.
Interior Design and Composition: MWdesign, Inc.

Printed in China

Last digit is the print number: 9 8

RISK FACTORS FOR CORONARY ARTERY DISEASE

Cardiovascular Disease Risk Factors		
Non-modifiable (Fixed) Factors	**Modifiable Factors**	**Contributing Factors**
• Heredity	• High blood pressure	• Stress
• Race	• Elevated serum cholesterol levels	• Inflammatory markers
• Gender	• Tobacco use	• Psychosocial factors
• Age	• Diabetes • Physical inactivity • Obesity • Metabolic syndrome	• Alcohol intake

Blood Pressure Values in Adults*

Category	Systolic blood pressure (in mm Hg)	Diastolic blood pressure (in mm Hg)
Normal	Less than 120	Less than 80
Prehypertension	120 to 139	80 to 89
Stage 1 high blood pressure	140 to 159	90 to 99
Stage 2 high blood pressure	160 or higher	100 or higher

From the National Heart Lung and Blood Institute:
High blood pressure,
www.nhlbi.nih.gov/health/dci/Diseases/Hbp/HBP_WhatIs.html. Accessed 5/15/2005.

* For adults 18 and older who:
  • Are not on medicine for high bloodpressure
  • Are not having a short-term serious illness
  • Do not have other conditions such as diabetes and kidney disease

SUDDEN CARDIAC DEATH

• Cardiopulmonary (cardiac) arrest is the absence of cardiac mechanical activity, confirmed by the absence of a detectable pulse, unresponsiveness, and apnea or agonal, gasping breathing.

• Sudden cardiac death (SCD) is an unexpected death due to a cardiac cause that occurs either immediately or within 1 hour of the onset of symptoms.

  ‣ Some victims of SCD have no warning signs of the impending event. For others, warning signs may be present up to 1 hour before the actual arrest.

  ‣ Because of irreversible brain damage and dependence upon life support, some patients may live days to weeks after the cardiac arrest before biological death occurs. These factors influence interpretation of the 1 hour definition of sudden cardiac death.[1]

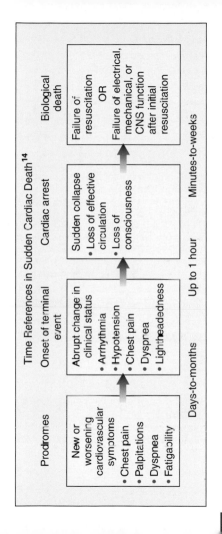

Time References in Sudden Cardiac Death[14]

Prodromes	Onset of terminal event	Cardiac arrest	Biological death
New or worsening cardiovascular symptoms • Chest pain • Palpitations • Dyspnea • Fatigability	Abrupt change in clinical status • Arrhythmia • Hypotension • Chest pain • Dyspnea • Lightheadedness	Sudden collapse • Loss of effective circulation • Loss of consciousness	Failure of resuscitation OR Failure of electrical, mechanical, or CNS function after initial resuscitation
Days-to-months	Up to 1 hour	Minutes-to-weeks	

CARDIAC ARREST RHYTHMS

Shockable rhythms

- Ventricular tachycardia (VT)
- Ventricular fibrillation (VF)

Nonshockable rhythms

- Asystole
- Pulseless electrical activity (PEA)

CHAIN OF SURVIVAL

The Chain of Survival represents the ideal series of events that should take place immediately after the recognition of the onset of sudden illness. The chain consists of five key steps that are interrelated. Following these steps gives the victim the best chance of surviving a heart attack or sudden cardiac arrest. The links in the chain of survival for adults include early recognition and activation, early CPR, early defibrillation, early advanced life support (ALS), and integrated post-cardiac arrest care.

BASIC LIFE SUPPORT

COMPONENTS OF BASIC LIFE SUPPORT

Recognition of signs of:

- Cardiac arrest
- Heart attack
- Stroke
- Foreign-body airway obstruction (FBAO)

Relief of FBAO
Cardiopulmonary resuscitation (CPR)
Defibrillation with an automated external defibrillator (AED)

Phases of CPR			
Phase	Phase Name	Time from VF arrest	Important intervention
1	Electrical phase	From time of arrest to about the first 5 min after arrest	Electrical therapy
2	Circulatory (hemodynamic) phase	About 5 min to 15 min after arrest	CPR before electrical therapy
3	Metabolic phase	After about 15 min	Therapeutic hypothermia

COMPONENTS OF ADVANCED CARDIAC CARE

- Basic life support
- Advanced airway management
- Ventilation support
- ECG/dysrhythmia recognition
- 12-lead ECG interpretation
- Vascular access and fluid resuscitation
- Electrical therapy including defibrillation, synchronized cardioversion, and pacing
- Giving medications
- Coronary artery bypass, stent insertion, angioplasty, intraaortic balloon pump therapy

Summary of Treatment for Adult, Child, Infant Choking, and CPR

CPR/Rescue Breathing	Infant	Child	Adult/Older Child
Age	Under 1 year	1 to about 12 to 14 years	More than 12 to 14 years
Level of Responsiveness	Establish unresponsiveness, tap and ask loudly, "Are you okay?"		
Check for breathing	If normal breathing is present, CPR is not needed. If the victim is unresponsive and not breathing (or only gasping), ask someone to activate the emergency response system and get a defibrillator.*		
C = Circulation	**Brachial**	**Carotid**	**Carotid**
Check pulse	Pulse present, support airway and breathing. No pulse, start compressions	Pulse present, support airway and breathing. No pulse, start compressions, call for AED	Pulse present, support airway and breathing. No pulse, start compressions, call for AED
Check landmarks	Just below nipple line	Just below nipple line	Just below nipple line
Compress chest with	2 fingers (1 rescuer) or 2 thumbs encircling chest (2 rescuers)	Heel of 1 hand or as for adult	Heel of 1 hand, other hand on top
Compression depth	At least 1/3 the anterior-posterior diameter of the chest (about 1.5 in [4 cm])	At least 1/3 the anterior-posterior diameter of the chest (about 2 in [5 cm])	At least 2 in (5 cm)
Compression rate	At least 100/min	At least 100/min	At least 100/min
Compression/ventilation ratio	1 rescuer = 30:2 2 rescuers = 15:2	1 rescuer = 30:2 2 rescuers = 15:2	1 or 2 rescuers = 30:2

6

CPR/Rescue Breathing	Infant	Child	Adult/Older Child
A = Airway			
B = Breathing	Deliver 2 breaths; each breath should take about 1 sec. Make sure the breaths are effective (the chest rises). If the chest does not rise, reposition the head, make a better seal, and try again. Avoid excessive ventilation (too many breaths, too large a volume).		
D = Defibrillation, if necessary	CPR for 5 cycles, recheck pulse. If no pulse, continue CPR. Recheck pulse every 5 cycles (about every 2 minutes).	If witnessed arrest, use AED. Power on AED, apply pads. Analyze rhythm, shock if indicated using pediatric pads/cable system	If witnessed arrest, use AED. Power on AED, apply pads. Analyze rhythm, shock if indicated
	Manual defibrillator preferred. If a manual defibrillator is not available, an AED equipped with a pediatric attenuator is desirable. If neither is available, use a standard AED.	Use AED equipped with a pediatric attenuator, if available. If unavailable, use standard AED.	Use standard AED.
	If shock advised, clear victim, give 1 shock, immediately resume CPR for 5 cycles, then reanalyze rhythm. Shock delivery should ideally occur as soon as possible after compressions. If no shock advised, immediately resume CPR.		

*A lone rescuer should perform 5 cycles of CPR (about 30 compressions and 2 breaths for about 2 min) before leaving an infant or child victim (or adult victim of presumed asphyxial arrest, such as drowning) to activate the emergency response system and obtain an AED.

INITIAL GOALS OF POST-CARDIAC ARREST CARE*

- Provide cardiorespiratory support to optimize tissue perfusion—especially to the heart, brain, and lungs (the organs most affected by cardiac arrest).

- Transport of the out-of-hospital post-cardiac arrest patient to an appropriate facility capable of providing comprehensive post–cardiac arrest care including acute coronary interventions, neurological care, goal-directed critical care, and hypothermia.

- Transport of the in-hospital post-cardiac arrest patient to a critical care unit capable of providing comprehensive post–cardiac arrest care.

- Attempt to identify the precipitating cause of the arrest, start specific treatment if necessary, and take actions to prevent recurrence.

*Peberdy MA, Callaway CW, Neumar RW, et al. Part 9: post–cardiac arrest care: 2010 American Heart Association Guidelines for Cardiopulmonary Resuscitation and Emergency Cardiovascular Care. *Circulation.* 2010;122(suppl 3):S768 –S786.

POSSIBLE TREATABLE CAUSES
OF CARDIAC EMERGENCIES

PATCH-4-MD

Pulmonary embolism — anticoagulants? surgery?

Acidosis — ventilation, correct acid-base disturbances

Tension pneumothorax — needle decompression

Cardiac tamponade — pericardiocentesis

Hypovolemia — replace volume

Hypoxia — ensure adequate oxygenation and ventilation

Heat / cold (hyperthermia/hypothermia) — cooling/warming methods

Hypo-/hyperkalemia (and other electrolytes) — monitor serum glucose levels closely, correct electrolyte disturbances

Myocardial infarction — reperfusion therapy

Drug overdose / accidents — antidote/specific thorapy

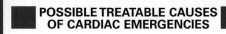

POSSIBLE TREATABLE CAUSES OF CARDIAC EMERGENCIES

Five Hs and Five Ts

Hypovolemia	**T**amponade, cardiac
Hypoxia	**T**ension pneumothorax
Hypothermia	**T**hrombosis: lungs *(massive pulmonary embolism)*
Hypo-/Hyperkalemia	**T**hrombosis: heart *(acute coronary syndromes)*
Hydrogen ion *(acidosis)*	**T**ablets/toxins: drug overdose

AIRWAY MANAGEMENT AND VENTILATION

Airway

Oxygen Percentage Delivery by Device

Device	Approximate Inspired Oxygen Concentration	Liter Flow (Liters/Minute)
Nasal Cannula	22% to 45%	0.25 to 8
Simple Face Mask	35% to 60%	5 to 10
Partial Rebreather Mask	35% to 60%	Typically 6 to 10 to prevent bag collapse
Nonrebreather Mask	60% to 80%	Typically 10 to prevent bag collapse

Manual Airway Maneuvers

	Head-tilt/chin-lift	Jaw thrust without head-tilt
Indications	Unresponsive patient • No mechanism for cervical spine injury • Unable to protect own airway	Unresponsive patient • Possible cervical spine injury • Unable to protect own airway
Contraindications	• Awake patient • Possible cervical spine injury	• Awake patient
Advantages	• Simple to preform • No equipment required • Noninvasive	• No equipment required • Noninvasive
Disadvantages	• Does not protect lower airway from aspiration • May cause spinal movement	• Difficult to maintain • Second rescuer needed for bag-valve-mask ventilation • Does not protect lower airway from aspiration • May cause spinal movement

Mouth-to-Mask Ventilation

Inspired Oxygen Concentration	• Without supplemental oxygen equals about 16% to 17% (exhaled air) • Mouth-to-mask breathing combined with supplemental oxygen at a minimum flow rate of 10 L/min equals about 50%
Advantages	• Aesthetically more acceptable than mouth-to-mouth ventilation • Easy to teach and learn • Physical barrier between the rescuer and the patient's nose, mouth, and secretions • Reduces (but does not prevent) the risk of exposure to infectious disease • Use of a one-way valve at the ventilation port decreases exposure to patient's exhaled air • If the patient resumes spontaneous breathing, the mask can be used as a simple face mask to deliver 40% to 60% oxygen by giving supplemental oxygen through the oxygen inlet on the mask (if so equipped). • Can deliver a greater tidal volume with mouth-to-mask ventilation than with a bag-mask device • Rescuer can feel the compliance of the patient's lungs (Compliance refers to the resistance of the patient's lung tissue to ventilation)
Disadvantages	• Rescuer fatigue • Possible gastric distention

Oral and Nasal Airways

	Oral Airway	Nasal Airway
Indications	• Help maintain an open airway in an unresponsive patient who is not intubated • Help maintain an open airway in an unresponsive patient with no gag reflex who is being ventilated with a bag-mask or other positive-pressure device • May be used as a bite block after insertion of a tracheal tube or orogastric tube	• To aid in maintaining an open airway when use of an oral airway is contraindicated or impossible • Trismus (spasm of the muscles used to grind, crush, and chew food) • Biting • Clenched jaws or teeth
Contraindications	• Responsive patient	• Severe craniofacial trauma • Patient intolerance
Sizing	• Corner of mouth to tip of earlobe or angle of jaw	• Tip of nose to angle of the jaw or the tip of the ear
Advantages	• Positions the tongue forward and away from the back of the throat • Easily placed	• Provides an open airway • Tolerated by responsive patients • Does not require mouth to be open

Disadvantages	• Does not protect the lower airway from aspiration • May produce vomiting if used in a responsive or semi-responsive patient with a gag reflex	• Does not protect the lower airway from aspiration • Improper technique may result in severe bleeding • Resulting epistaxis may be difficult to control • Suctioning through the device is difficult • Although tolerated by most responsive and semi-responsive patients, can stimulate the gag reflex in sensitive patients, precipitating laryngospasm and vomiting
Precautions	• Use of the device does not eliminate the need for maintaining proper head position	• Use of the device does not eliminate the need for maintaining proper head position

Bag-Mask Ventilation	
Advantages	• Provides a means for delivery of an oxygen enriched mixture to the patient • Conveys a sense of compliance of patient's lungs to the bag-mask operator • Provides a means for immediate ventilatory support • Can be used with the spontaneously breathing patient as well as the non-breathing patient
Disadvantages	• Requires practice to use effectively • Delivery of inadequate tidal volume • Rescuer fatigue • Possible gastric distention

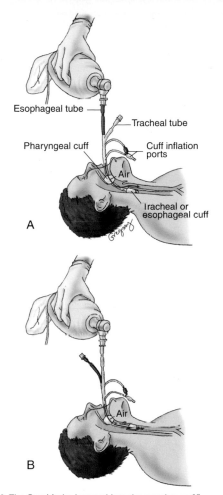

Esophageal tube

Tracheal tube

Pharyngeal cuff

Cuff inflation ports

Air

Tracheal or esophageal cuff

A

Air

B

A, The Combitube inserted into the esophagus.[16]
B, The Combitube inserted into the trachea.[16]

Combitube

Indications	• Difficult face mask fit (beards, absence of teeth) • Patient in whom intubation has been unsuccessful and ventilation is difficult • Patient in whom airway management is necessary but the healthcare provider is untrained in the technique of visualized orotracheal intubation
Contraindications	• Patient with an intact gag reflex • Patient with known or suspected esophageal disease • Patient known to have ingested a caustic substance • Suspected upper airway obstruction due to laryngeal foreign body or pathology • Patient less than 4 feet tall
Advantages	• Minimal training and retraining required Visualization of the upper airway or use of special equipment not required for insertion • Reasonable technique for use in suspected neck injury since the head does not need to be hyperextended • Because of the oropharyngeal balloon, the need for a face mask is eliminated • Can provide an open airway with either esophageal or tracheal placement • If placed in the esophagus, allows suctioning of gastric contents without interruption of ventilation • Reduces risk of aspiration of gastric contents

Combitube—cont'd	
Disadvantages	• Proximal port may be occluded with secretions • Proper identification of tube location may be difficult, leading to ventilation through the wrong lumen • Soft tissue trauma due to rigidity of tube • Impossible to suction the trachea when the tube is in the esophagus • Esophageal or tracheal trauma due to poor insertion technique or use of wrong size device • Damage to the cuffs by the patient's teeth during insertion • Inability to insert due to limited mouth opening

Laryngeal Mask Airway

Indications	• Difficult face mask fit (beards, absence of teeth) • Patient in whom intubation has been unsuccessful and ventilation is difficult • Patient in whom airway management is necessary but the healthcare provider is untrained in the technique of visualized orotracheal intubation • Many elective surgical procedures (i.e., minimal soft tissue trauma with less patient discomfort and relatively short periods of anesthesia)
Contraindications	• Healthcare provider untrained in use of Laryngeal Mask Airway (LMA) • Contraindicated if a risk of aspiration exists (i.e., patients with full stomachs)
Advantages	• Can be quickly inserted to provide ventilation when bag-mask ventilation is not sufficient and tracheal intubation cannot be readily accomplished • Tidal volume delivered may be greater when using the LMA than with face mask ventilation • Less gastric insufflation than with bag-mask ventilation • Provides ventilation equivalent to the tracheal tube • Training simpler than with tracheal intubation • Unaffected by anatomic factors (e.g., beard, absence of teeth) • No risk of esophageal or bronchial intubation • When compared to tracheal intubation, less potential for trauma from direct laryngoscopy and tracheal intubation • Less coughing, laryngeal spasm, sore throat, and voice changes than with tracheal intubation

Laryngeal Mask Airway—cont'd

Disadvantages	• Does not provide protection against aspiration • Cannot be used if the mouth cannot be opened more than 0.6 in (1.5 cm) • May not be effective when respiratory anatomy is abnormal (i.e., abnormal oropharyngeal anatomy or the presence of pathology is likely to result in a poor mask fit) • May be difficult to provide adequate ventilation if high airway pressures are required

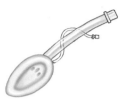

A

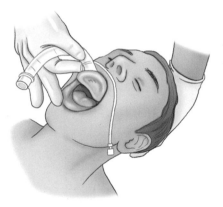

B

The laryngeal mask airway (LMA). **A**, An LMA with the cuff inflated. **B**, LMA placement into the pharynx. **C**, LMA placement using the index finger as a guide. **D**, LMA in place with cuff overlying pharynx.[17]

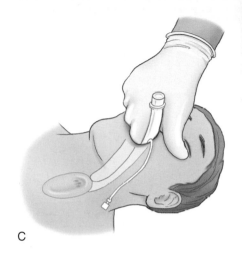

C

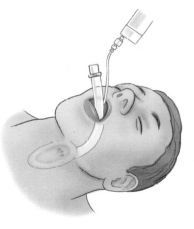

D

Tracheal Intubation

Indications	• Inability of the patient to protect his or her own airway due to the absence of protective reflexes (e.g., coma, respiratory and/or cardiac arrest) • Inability of the rescuer to ventilate the unresponsive patient with less invasive methods • Present or impending airway obstruction/respiratory failure (e.g., inhalation injury, severe asthma, exacerbation of chronic obstructive pulmonary disease, severe pulmonary edema, severe flail chest or pulmonary contusion) • When prolonged ventilatory support is required
Contraindications	• Healthcare provider untrained in tracheal intubation
Advantages	• Isolates the airway • Keeps the airway open • Reduces the risk of aspiration • Ensures delivery of a high concentration of oxygen • Permits suctioning of the trachea • Provides a route for administration of some medications (see IV/Meds chapter) • Ensures delivery of a selected tidal volume to maintain lung inflation
Disadvantages	• Considerable training and experience required; retraining may be needed to ensure competency • Special equipment needed • Bypasses physiologic function of upper airway (e.g., warming, filtering, humidifying of inhaled air) • Requires direct visualization of vocal cords

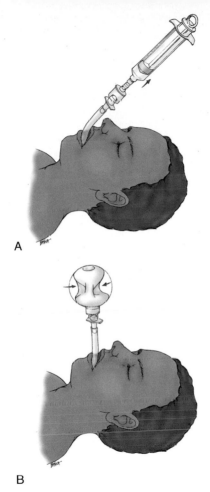

A

B

Esophageal detector device. **A**, Syringe. **B**, Bulb.[18]

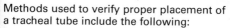

CONFIRMING TRACHEAL TUBE PLACEMENT

Methods used to verify proper placement of a tracheal tube include the following:

- Visualizing the passage of the tracheal tube between the vocal cords
- Auscultating the presence of bilateral breath sounds
- Confirming the absence of sounds over the epigastrium during ventilation
- Adequate chest rise with each ventilation
- Absence of vocal sounds after placement of the tracheal tube
- End-tidal carbon dioxide measurement (waveform capnography preferred)
- Verification of tube placement by an esophageal detector device
- Chest radiograph

RHYTHM RECOGNITION

ECGs

Summary of Standard Limb Leads

Lead	Positive Electrode	Negative Electrode	Heart Surface Viewed
Lead I	Left arm	Right arm	Lateral
Lead II	Left leg	Right arm	Inferior
Lead III	Left leg	Left arm	Inferior

Summary of Augmented Leads

Lead	Positive Electrode	Heart Surface Viewed
Lead aVR	Right arm	None
Lead aVL	Left arm	Lateral
Lead aVF	Left leg	Inferior

Summary of Standard Limb Leads

Lead	Positive Electrode Position	Heart Surface Viewed
Lead V_1	Right side of sternum, 4th intercostal space	Septum
Lead V_2	Left side of sternum, 4th intercostal space	Septum
Lead V_3	Midway between V_2 and V_4	Anterior
Lead V_4	Left midclavicular line, 5th intercostal space	Anterior
Lead V_5	Left anterior axillary line at same level as V_4	Lateral
Lead V_6	Left midaxillary line at same level as V_4	Lateral

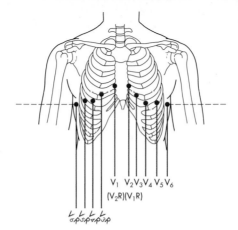

Placement of the left and right chest leads.[19]

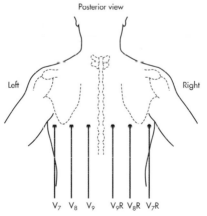

Posterior chest lead placement.[20]

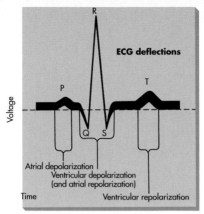

ECG waveforms—P, QRS, and T.[21]

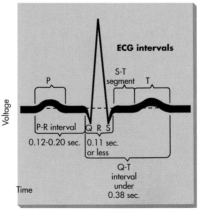

ECG segments and intervals—PR interval, QRS duration, ST-segment, QT interval.[21]

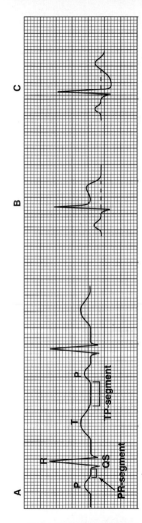

The TP-segment. **A,** The TP-segment is used as the baseline from which to determine the presence of ST-segment elevation or depression. **B,** ST-segment elevation. **C,** ST-segment depression.[22]

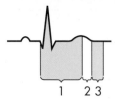

Refractory periods. **1,** The absolute refractory period, **2,** Relative refractory period. **3,** The supernormal period.[23]

TOO FAST RHYTHMS

NARROW-QRS TACHYCARDIAS

Sinus Tachycardia

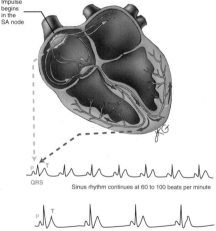

Impulse begins in the SA node

Sinus rhythm continues at 60 to 100 beats per minute

Sinus bradycardia continues at less than 60 beats per minute

Sinus tachycardia continues faster than 100 beats per minute

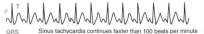

Sinus rhythm, sinus bradycardia, and sinus tachycardia.[24]

Sinus Tachycardia

Rate	101 to 180 bpm
Rhythm	Regular
P waves	Uniform in appearance, positive (upright) in lead II, one precedes each QRS complex; at very fast rates it may be difficult to distinguish a P wave from a T wave
PR interval	0.12-0.20 second and constant from beat to beat
QRS duration	0.11 second or less unless an intraventricular conduction delay exists

Atrial Tachycardia

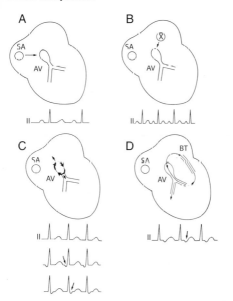

Supraventricular tachycardias. **A**, Normal sinus rhythm. **B**, Atrial tachycardia. **C**, AV nodal reentrant tachycardia (AVNRT). **D**, AV reentrant tachycardia (AVRT).[25]

Atrial Tachycardia (AT)

Rate	150 to 250 bpm
Rhythm	Regular
P waves	One positive P wave precedes each QRS complex in lead II but the P waves differ in shape from sinus P waves. With rapid rates, it is difficult to distinguish P waves from T waves.
PR interval	May be shorter or longer than normal and may be difficult to measure because P waves may be hidden in T waves
QRS duration	0.11 second or less unless an intraventricular conduction delay exists

AV Nodal Reentrant Tachycardia (AVNRT)

Rate	150 to 250 bpm; typically 170 to 250 bpm
Rhythm	Ventricular rhythm is usually very regular
P waves	P waves are often hidden in the QRS complex. If the ventricles are stimulated first and then the atria, a negative (inverted) P wave will appear after the QRS in leads II, III, and aVF. When the atria are depolarized after the ventricles, the P wave typically distorts the end of the QRS complex.
PR interval	P waves are not seen before the QRS complex, therefore the PR interval is not measurable
QRS duration	0.11 second or less unless an intraventricular conduction delay exists

AV Reentrant Tachycardia (AVRT)

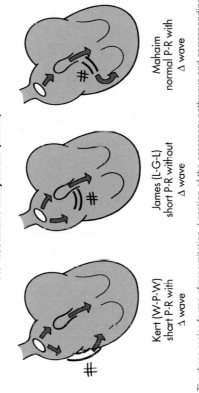

Kert (W-P-W)
short P-R with
Δ wave

James (L-G-L)
short P-R without
Δ wave

Mahaim
normal P-R with
Δ wave

The three major forms of preexcitation. Location of the accessory pathways and corresponding ECG characteristics.

V_3

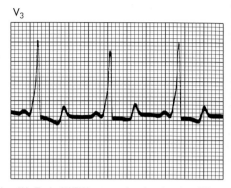

Lead V_3. Typical WPW pattern showing the short PR interval, delta wave, wide QRS complex and secondary ST, and T-wave changes.[27]

Wolff-Parkinson-White (WPW) Syndrome	
Rate	Usually 60-100 bpm, if the underlying rhythm is sinus in origin
Rhythm	Regular, unless associated with atrial fibrillation
P waves	Upright in lead II unless WPW is associated with atrial fibrillation
PR interval	If P waves are observed, less than 0.12 second because the impulse travels very quickly across the accessory pathway, bypassing the normal delay in the AV node
QRS duration	Usually greater than 0.12 second. Slurred upstroke of the QRS complex (delta wave) may be seen in one or more leads.

Junctional Tachycardia[28]

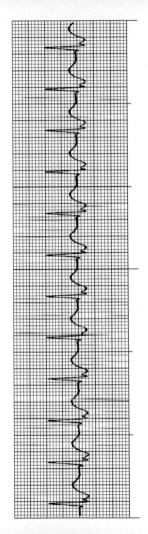

Junctional Tachycardia

Rate	101-180 bpm
Rhythm	Very regular
P waves	May occur before, during, or after the QRS. If visible, the P wave is inverted in leads II, III, and aVF
PR interval	If a P wave occurs before the QRS, the PR interval will usually be less than or equal to 0.12 second. If no P wave occurs before the QRS, there will be no PR interval.
QRS duration	0.11 second or less unless an intraventricular conduction delay exists.

WIDE-QRS TACHYCARDIAS

Intraventricular Conduction Defects

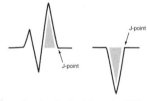

Move from the J-point back into the QRS complex and determine whether the terminal portion (last 0.04 second) of the QRS complex is a positive (upright) or negative (downward) deflection. If the two criteria for bundle branch block are met and the terminal portion of the QRS is positive, a right bundle branch block (BBB) is most likely present. If the terminal portion of the QRS is negative, a left BBB is most likely present.[29]

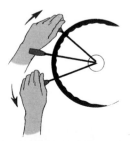

Differentiating right versus left BBB. The "turn signal theory" — right is up, left is down.[29]

Monomorphic VT

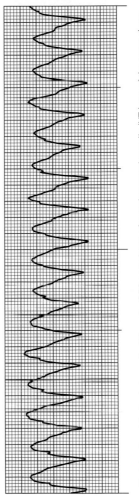

Sustained ventricular tachycardia. When the QRS complexes of ventricular tachycardia (VT) are of the same shape and amplitude, the rhythm is called *monomorphic VT*.[30]

Monomorphic Ventricular Tachycardia

Rate	101-250 bpm
Rhythm	Essentially regular
P waves	Usually not seen; if present, they have no set relationship to the QRS complexes appearing between them at a rate different from that of the VT
PR interval	None
QRS duration	Greater than 0.12 second; often difficult to differentiate between the QRS and T wave

IRREGULAR TACHYCARDIAS

Multifocal Atrial Tachycardia

Rate	Ventricular rate is greater than 100 bpm
Rhythm	May be irregular as the pacemaker site shifts from the SA node to ectopic atrial locations and the AV junction
P waves	Size, shape, and direction may change from beat to beat; at least three different P wave configurations (seen in the same lead) are required for a diagnosis of wandering atrial pacemaker or multifocal atrial tachycardia
PR interval	Variable
QRS duration	0.11 second or less unless an intraventricular conduction delay exists

Multifocal Atrial Tachycardia (MAT)[31]

Atrial Flutter

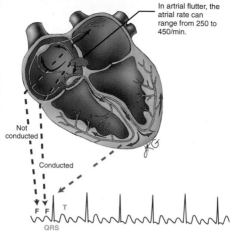

In atrial flutter, the atrial rate can range from 250 to 450/min.

Not conducted

Conducted

F F T
QRS

Atrial flutter. *F*, Flutter wave.[32]

Atrial Flutter	
Rate	In type I atrial flutter (also called typical rapid atrial flutter), the atrial rate ranges from 250 to 350 bpm. In type II atrial flutter (also called atypical or very rapid atrial flutter), the atrial rate ranges from 350 to 450 bpm.
Rhythm	Atrial regular, ventricular regular or irregular depending on AV conduction/blockade
P waves	No identifiable P waves; saw-toothed "flutter" waves are present
PR interval	Not measurable
QRS duration	Usually less than 0.11 second but may be widened if flutter waves are buried in the QRS complex or an intraventricular conduction delay exists

Atrial Fibrillation

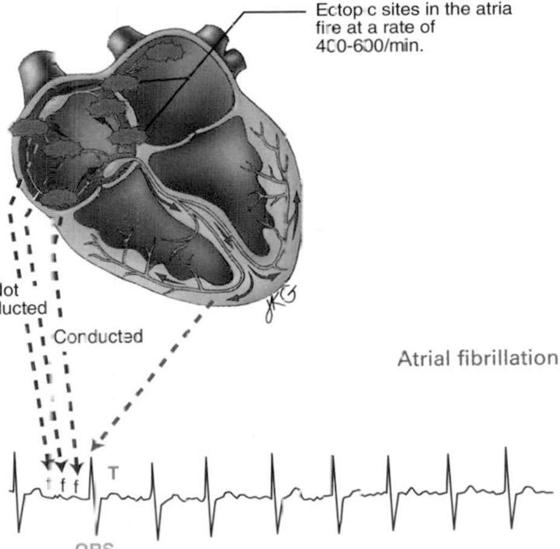

Ectopic sites in the atria fire at a rate of 400-600/min.

Conducted

Not conducted

Atrial fibrillation. *f*, Fibrillatory wave.[32]

Only some of the atrial impulses are conducted through the AV node.

Atrial impulses produce an erratic wavy baseline before the QRS complexes.

T

QRS

Atrial Fibrillation

Rate	Atrial rate usually greater than 400-600 bpm; ventricular rate variable
Rhythm	Ventricular rhythm usually irregularly irregular
P waves	No identifiable P waves; fibrillatory waves present. Erratic, wavy baseline.
PR interval	Not measurable
QRS duration	Usually less than 0.11 second but may be widened if an intraventricular conduction delay exists

Polymorphic Ventricular Tachycardia

Rate	150 to 300 bpm, typically 200-250 bpm
Rhythm	May be regular or irregular
P waves	None
PR interval	None
QRS duration	Greater than 0.12 sec; gradual alteration in amplitude and direction of the QRS complexes; a typical cycle consists of 5 to 20 QRS complexes

Polymorphic Ventricular Tachycardia

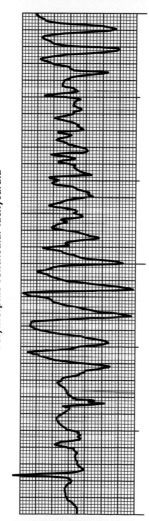

When the QRS complexes of ventricular tachycardia (VT) vary in shape and amplitude, the rhythm is termed *polymorphic VT*.[3]

SINUS BRADYCARDIA

Sinus Bradycardia	
Rate	Less than 60 bpm
Rhythm	Regular
P waves	Uniform in appearance, positive (upright) in lead II, one precedes each QRS complex
PR interval	0.12-0.20 second and constant from beat to beat
QRS duration	0.11 second or less unless an intraventricular conduction delay exists

Sinus Bradycardia[34]

JUNCTIONAL RHYTHM

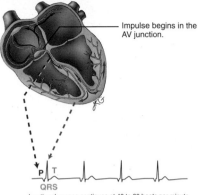

Impulse begins in the AV junction.

P T QRS

Junctional escape continues at 40 to 60 beats per minute.

P T QRS

Accelerated junctional rhythm continues at 60 to 100 beats per minute.

P T QRS

Junctional tachycardia continues at 100 to 180 beats per minute.

Junctional rhythms.[35]

Junctional Escape Rhythm	
Rate	40 to 60 bpm
Rhythm	Very regular
P waves	May occur before, during, or after the QRS. If visible, the P wave is inverted in leads II, III, and aVF.
PR interval	If a P wave occurs before the QRS, the PR interval will usually be less than or equal to 0.12 second. If no P wave occurs before the QRS, there will be no PR interval.
QRS duration	0.11 second or less unless an intraventricular conduction delay exists.

Ventricular Escape Rhythm[36]

Ventricular Escape (Idioventricular) Rhythm

Rate	20 to 40 bpm
Rhythm	Essentially regular
P waves	Usually absent or, with retrograde conduction to the atria, may appear after the QRS (usually upright in the ST-segment or T wave)
PR interval	None
QRS duration	Greater than 0.12 second, T wave frequently in opposite direction of the QRS complex

FIRST-DEGREE AV BLOCK

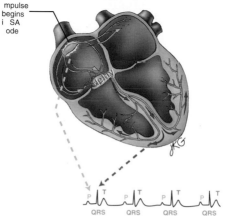

mpulse
begins
i SA
ode

delay

P   T   P   T   P   T   P   T
QRS   QRS   QRS   QRS

First-degree atrioventricular (AV) block.[37]

First-Degree AV Block	
Rate	Usually within normal range, but depends on underlying rhythm
Rhythm	Regular
P waves	Normal in size and shape, one positive (upright) P wave before each QRS in leads II, III, and aVF
PR interval	Prolonged (greater than 0.20 second) but constant
QRS duration	0.11 second or less unless an intraventricular conduction delay exists

SECOND-DEGREE AV BLOCK–TYPE I
(WENCKEBACH, MOBITZ TYPE I)[37]

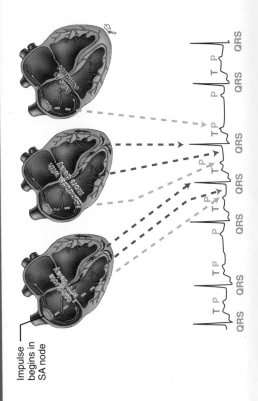

Impulse begins in SA node

Second-Degree AV Block–Type I

Rate	Atrial rate is greater than the ventricular rate
Rhythm	Atrial regular (P's plot through on time), ventricular irregular
P waves	Normal in size and shape. Some P waves are not followed by a QRS complex (more P's than QRSs).
PR interval	**Lengthens with each cycle** (although lengthening may be very slight), until a P wave appears without a QRS complex. The PRI *after* the nonconducted beat is shorter than the interval preceding the nonconducted beat.
QRS duration	Usually 0.11 second or less but is periodically dropped.

SECOND-DEGREE AV BLOCK–TYPE II (MOBITZ TYPE II)

Second-Degree AV Block–Type II

Rate	Atrial rate is greater than the ventricular rate. Ventricular rate is often slow.
Rhythm	Atrial regular (P's plot through on time), ventricular irregular.
P waves	Normal in size and shape. Some P waves are not followed by a QRS complex (more P's than QRSs).
PR interval	Within normal limits or slightly prolonged but **constant** for the conducted beats. There may be some shortening of the PR interval that follows a nonconducted P wave.
QRS duration	Usually 0.11 second or greater, periodically absent after P waves.

Second Degree AV Block–Type II[38]

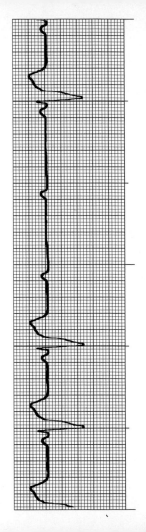

Second-Degree AV Block 2:1 Conduction (2:1 AV Block)

Rate	Atrial rate is twice the ventricular rate
Rhythm	Atrial regular (P's plot through). Ventricular regular.
P waves	Normal in size and shape; every other P wave is followed by a QRS complex (more P's than QRSs)
PR interval	Constant
QRS duration	Within normal limits, if the block occurs above the bundle of His (probably type I); wide if the block occurs below the bundle of His (probably type II); absent after every other P wave.

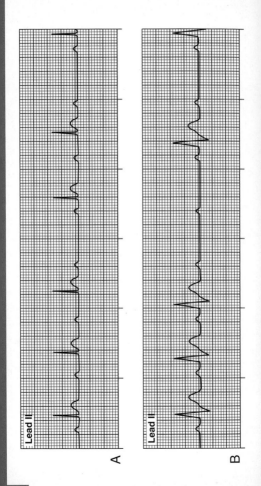

Lead II

A

Lead II

B

56

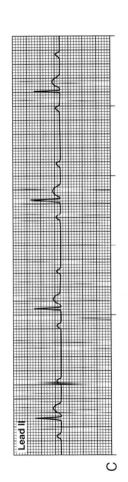

Types of second-degree AV block. **A,** Second-degree AV block type I; **B,** second-degree AV block type II; **C,** 2:1 AV block.[39]

C

THIRD-DEGREE AV BLOCK

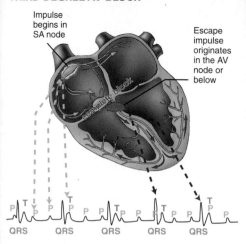

Third-degree AV block.[40]

Third-degree AV Block	
Rate	Atrial rate is greater than the ventricular rate. The ventricular rate is determined by the origin of the escape rhythm.
Rhythm	Atrial regular (P's plot through). Ventricular regular. There is no relationship between the atrial and ventricular rhythms.
P waves	Normal in size and shape.
PR interval	*None*—the atria and ventricles beat independently of each other, thus there is no true PR interval.
QRS duration	Narrow or wide depending on the location of the escape pacemaker and the condition of the intraventricular conduction system. Narrow = junctional pacemaker, wide = ventricular pacemaker.

Ventricular Fibrillation (VF)

Rate	Cannot be determined because there are no discernible waves or complexes to measure
Rhythm	Rapid and chaotic with no pattern or regularity
P waves	Not discernible
PR interval	Not discernible
QRS duration	Not discernible

Ventricular Fibrillation (VF)[41]

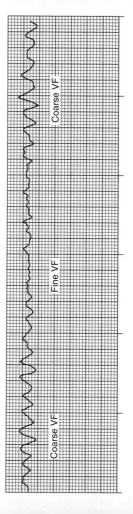

Coarse VF

Fine VF

Coarse VF

Coarse and fine ventricular fibrillation.

Ventricular Tachycardia (VT).[42]

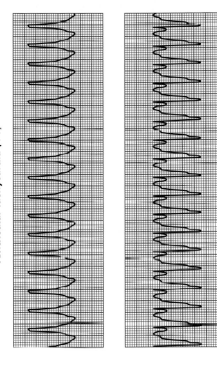

Ventricular Tachycardia

Rate	101-250 bpm
Rhythm	Essentially regular
P waves	Usually not seen; if present, they have no set relationship to the QRS complexes appearing between them at a rate different from that of the VT
PR interval	None
QRS duration	Greater than 0.12 second; often difficult to differentiate between the QRS and T wave

ASYSTOLE (CARDIAC STANDSTILL)

Asystole

Rate	Ventricular usually not discernible but atrial activity may be observed ("P wave" asystole)
Rhythm	Ventricular not discernible, atrial may be discernible
P waves	Usually not discernible
PR interval	Not measurable
QRS duration	Absent

Asystole[43]

"P-Wave" Asystole[44]

PULSELESS ELECTRICAL ACTIVITY

Pulseless electrical activity (PEA) is a clinical situation, not a specific dysrhythmia. PEA exists when organized electrical activity (other than VT) is observed on the cardiac monitor but the patient is unresponsive, not breathing, and a pulse cannot be felt.

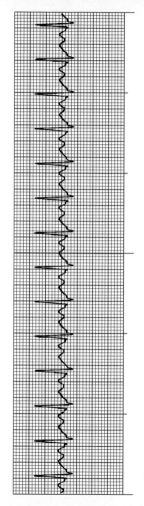

The rhythm shown is a sinus tachycardia; however, if no pulse is associated with the rhythm, the clinical situation is termed pulseless electrical activity (PEA).[44]

DEFIBRILLATION

Defibrillation is delivery of an electrical current across the heart muscle over a very brief period to terminate an abnormal heart rhythm. Defibrillation is also called *unsynchronized countershock,* or *asynchronous countershock,* because the delivery of current has no relationship to the cardiac cycle. Indications for defibrillation include sustained polymorphic VT, pulseless VT, and VF.

Defibrillation does not "jump start" the heart. The shock attempts to deliver a uniform electrical current of sufficient intensity to depolarize ventricular cells (including fibrillating cells) at the same time, briefly stunning the heart. This provides an opportunity for the heart's natural pacemakers to resume normal activity. When the cells repolarize, the pacemaker with the highest degree of automaticity should assume responsibility for pacing the heart.

Manual defibrillation refers to the placement of paddles or pads on a patient's chest, interpretation of the patient's cardiac rhythm by a trained healthcare professional, and the healthcare professional's decision to deliver a shock (if indicated). *Automated external defibrillation* refers to the placement of paddles or pads on a patient's chest and interpretation of the patient's cardiac rhythm by the defibrillator's computerized analysis system. Depending on the type of automated external defibrillator (AED) used, the machine will deliver a shock (if a shockable rhythm is detected) or instruct the operator to deliver a shock.

TRANSTHORACIC RESISTANCE

Although the energy selected for defibrillation or cardioversion is expressed in joules, it is current that delivers energy to the patient and depolarizes the myocardium. *Impedance* refers to the resistance to the flow of current and is measured in ohms. *Transthoracic impedance* (resistance) refers to the natural resistance of the chest wall to the flow of current. Transthoracic resistance varies greatly. Factors known to affect transthoracic resistance include the following:

- Paddle/electrode size
- Paddle/electrode position
- Use of conductive material (when using handheld paddles)
- Paddle pressure (when using handheld paddles)
- Selected energy

MONOPHASIC DEFIBRILLATION

Pressing the charge button on a defibrillator charges the capacitor. Once the capacitor is charged and the shock control is pressed, voltage pushes a flow of electrons (current) to the patient by means of handheld paddles or combination pads. Current passes through the heart in "waveforms" that travel from one paddle/pad, through the chest, and back to the other paddle/pad over a brief period.

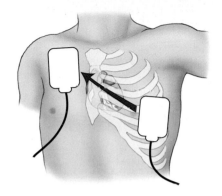

When a monophasic waveform is used, current passes through the heart in one direction.[45]

BIPHASIC DEFIBRILLATION

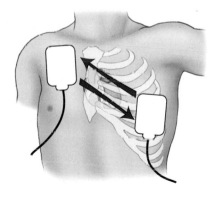

With biphasic waveforms, energy is delivered in two phases. The current moves in one direction for a specified period, stops, and then passes through the heart a second time in the opposite direction.[45]

AUTOMATED EXTERNAL DEFIBRILLATORS (AEDs)

An AED is an external defibrillator that has a computerized cardiac rhythm analysis system. AEDs are easy to use. Voice prompts and visual indicators guide the user through a series of steps that may include defibrillation.

When the adhesive electrodes are attached to the patient's chest, the AED examines and analyzes the patient's cardiac rhythm. Some AEDs require the operator to press an "analyze" control to initiate rhythm analysis whereas others automatically begin analyzing the patient's cardiac rhythm when the electrode pads are attached to the patient's chest. Safety filters check for false signals (e.g., radio transmissions, poor electrode contact, 60-cycle interference, loose electrodes).

When the AED analyzes the patient's cardiac rhythm, it "looks" at multiple features of the rhythm, including the QRS width, rate, and amplitude. If the AED detects a shockable rhythm, it charges the capacitors. In addition to VF, AEDs will recommend a shock for monomorphic VT and polymorphic VT. The preset rate for "shockable" VT varies depending on the AED. For instance, some manufacturers set the shockable VT rate (for adults) at greater than 150 beats/minute. Others set the rate at greater than 120 beats/minute.

If a shockable rhythm is detected by a fully automated AED, it will signal everyone to stand clear of the patient and then delivers a shock by means of the adhesive pads that were applied to the patient's chest.

If a shockable rhythm is detected by a semi-automated AED, it will instruct the AED operator (by means of voice prompts and visual signals) to press the shock control to deliver a shock.

Some AEDs:

- Can be configured to allow advanced life support personnel to switch to a manual mode, allowing more decision-making control
- Have CPR pads available that are equipped with a sensor. The sensor detects the depth of chest compressions. If the depth of chest compressions is inadequate, the machine provides voice prompts to the rescuer.
- Provide voice instructions in adult and infant-child CPR at the user's option. A metronome function encourages rescuers to perform chest compressions at the recommended rate of 100 compressions per minute.
- Are programmed to detect spontaneous movement by the patient or others.
- Have adapters available for many popular manual defibrillators, enabling the AED pads to remain on the patient when patient care is transferred
- Are equipped with a pediatric attenuator (pad-cable system or key). When the attenuator is attached to the AED, the machine recognizes the pediatric cable connection and automatically adjusts its defibrillation energy accordingly.

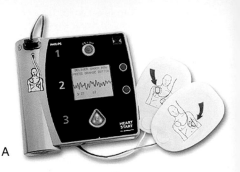

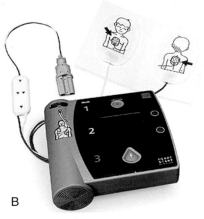

A, Automated external defibrillator (AED). **B,** This defibrillation pad and cable system reduces the energy delivered by a standard AED to that appropriate for a child.[46]

Use a standard AED for a patient who is unresponsive, apneic, pulseless, and 8 years of age or older. If the patient is between 1 and 8 years of age and a pediatric attenuator is unavailable for the AED, use a standard

AED. In infants, defibrillation with a manual defibrillator is preferred. If a manual defibrillator is not available, an AED equipped with a pediatric attenuator is desirable. If neither is available, use a standard AED.

Some AEDs can detect the patient's transthoracic resistance through the adhesive pads applied to the patient's chest. The AED automatically adjusts the voltage and length of the shock, thus customizing how the energy is delivered to that patient.

AED Operation

To operate an AED:

- Turn on the power.
- Attach the device.
- Analyze the rhythm.
- Deliver a shock if indicated and safe.

■ SYNCHRONIZED CARDIOVERSION ■

Synchronized cardioversion is a type of electrical therapy in which a shock is "timed" or "programmed" for delivery during the QRS complex. A synchronizing circuit in the machine searches for the highest (R wave deflection) or deepest (QS deflection) part of the QRS complex and delivers the shock a few milliseconds after this portion of the QRS. Delivery of a shock during this portion of the cardiac cycle reduces the potential for the delivery of current during the vulnerable period of the T wave (relative refractory period).

Synchronized cardioversion is used to treat rhythms that have a clearly identifiable QRS complex and a rapid ventricular rate (such as some narrow-QRS tachycardias and monomorphic VT).

Defibrillation and Cardioversion Summary

Type of Shock	Rhythm	Recommended Energy Levels
Defibrillation	• Pulseless ventricular tachycardia (VT)/ventricular fibrillation (VF) • Sustained polymorphic VT	Varies depending on device used • Biphasic defibrillator effective dose typically 120 J to 200 J • If effective dose range of defibrillator is unknown, consider using at the maximal dose • If using monophasic defibrillator, 360 J for all shocks
Cardioversion	Unstable narrow-QRS tachycardia	50 J to 100 J initially, increase in stepwise fashion if initial shock fails
	Unstable atrial flutter	50 J to 100 J initially, increase in stepwise fashion if initial shock fails
	Unstable atrial fibrillation	120 J to 200 J initially (biphasic), increase in stepwise fashion if initial shock fails; begin with 200 J if using monophasic energy and increase if unsuccessful
	Unstable monomorphic VT	100 J initially, reasonable to increase in stepwise fashion if initial shock fails

Synchronized cardioversion is not used to treat disorganized rhythms (such as polymorphic VT) or those that do not have a clearly identifiable QRS complex (such as VF).

DEFIBRILLATION AND SYNCHRONIZED CARDIOVERSION— SPECIAL CONSIDERATIONS

- Remove supplemental oxygen sources from the area of the patient's bed before defibrillation and cardioversion attempts and place them at least $3^{1}/_{2}$ to 4 feet from the patient's chest. Examples of supplemental oxygen sources include masks, nasal cannulae, resuscitation bags, and ventilator tubing. Case reports describe instances of fires ignited by sparks from poorly applied defibrillator paddles/pads in an oxygen-enriched atmosphere. Severe fires have resulted when ventilator tubing was disconnected from an endotracheal tube and then left next to the patient's head while defibrillation was attempted.

- To prevent fires during defibrillation attempts:
  - Be sure to use defibrillator paddles/pads of the appropriate size. Adult paddles/pads should be used for patients greater than 10 kg. Use pediatric paddles/pads for patients less than 10 kg.
  - Make sure there are no air pockets between the paddle/pads and the patient's skin. When applying combination pads to a patient's bare chest, press from one edge of the pad across the entire surface to remove all air.
  - When using handheld paddles, use appropriate conductive gel or disposable gel pads and apply firm, even pressure during defibrillation attempts.

- Keep monitoring electrodes and wires away from the area where defibrillator pads or combination pads will be placed. Contact may cause electrical arcing and patient skin burns during defibrillation or cardioversion.

- Remove transdermal patches, bandages, necklaces, or other materials from the sites used for paddle placement—do not attempt to defibrillate through them. Wipe residue from a medication patch or ointment from the patient's chest. Do not use alcohol or alcohol-based cleansers.

- If an unresponsive patient is lying in water or the patient's chest is covered with water, it may be reasonable to remove the victim from the water and quickly wipe the chest before applying the AED pads and attempting defibrillation.

- If the patient has a pacemaker or ICD, an AED may be used; but the AED pads should be placed at least 3 inches (8 cm) from the implanted device. If an ICD is in the process of delivering shocks to the patient, allow it about 30 to 60 seconds to complete its cycle.

TRANSCUTANEOUS PACING

- A pacemaker is an artificial pulse generator that delivers an electrical current to the heart to stimulate depolarization. Transcutaneous pacing (TCP) delivers pacing impulses to the heart using electrodes placed on the patient's chest. TCP is also called *temporary external pacing,* or *noninvasive pacing.*

- TCP is indicated for symptomatic bradycardias unresponsive to atropine therapy or when atropine is not immediately available or indicated. It may also be used as a "bridge" until transvenous pacing can be accomplished or the cause of the bradycardia is reversed (as in cases of drug overdose or hyperkalemia).

- Although TCP is a type of electrical therapy, the current delivered is considerably less than that used for cardioversion or defibrillation. The energy levels selected for cardioversion or defibrillation are indicated in joules. The stimulating current selected for TCP is indicated in milliamperes (mA). The range of output current of a transcutaneous pacemaker varies depending on the manufacturer.

PROCEDURE

- Pacing may be performed in either demand or nondemand (asynchronous) mode. The demand mode is used for most patients. When the pacemaker is in demand mode, pacing is inhibited when the pacemaker "senses" the patient's own (intrinsic) beats.
  - To detect the patient's own beats (QRS complexes), the pacemaker must be connected to ECG electrodes and an ECG cable. In addition, the QRS complexes must be of adequate size to be sensed by the pacemaker.
  - If the gain (ECG size) on the monitor is set too low to detect the patient's beats (or an ECG lead is off), the pacemaker produces pacing stimuli asynchronously. In other words, the pacemaker generates a pacing stimulus at the selected rate regardless of the patient's own rhythm.

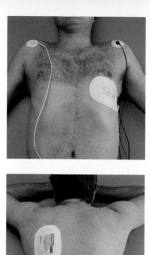

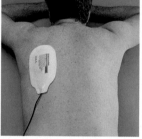

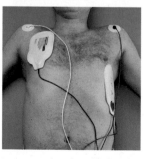

Transcutaneous pacing. **A** and **B**, Anterior-posterior pacing pad placement. **C**, Anterior-lateral pacing pad placement.[47]

- ▸ Place adhesive pacing pads on the patient's bare chest according to the manufacturer's instructions. The pads should fit completely on the patient's chest with a minimum of 1 inch of space between them. The pads should not overlap the sternum, spine, or scapula. In women, the anterior pacer pad is positioned *under* (not on) the left breast.
- Connect the patient to an ECG monitor, obtain a rhythm strip, and verify the presence of a paceable rhythm. Connect the pacing cable to the adhesive electrodes on the patient and the pulse generator.
- Turn the power on to the pacemaker and set the pacing rate. When TCP is used to treat a symptomatic bradycardia, the rate is set at a nonbradycardic rate, generally between 60 and 80 pulses per minute (ppm).

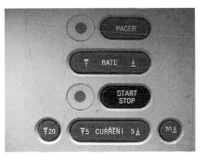

Transcutaneous pacemaker controls.[48]

- After the rate has been regulated, set the stimulating current. This control is usually labeled CURRENT, PACER OUTPUT, and/or mA. Increase the current slowly but steadily until capture is achieved. Sedation and/or analgesia may be needed to minimize the discomfort associated with this procedure (common with currents of 50 mA or more).

- Watch the cardiac monitor closely for *electrical* capture. This is usually evidenced by a wide QRS and a T wave that appears in a direction opposite the QRS. In some patients, electrical capture is not as obvious and appears only as a change in the shape of the QRS.

- Assess *mechanical* capture by checking the patient's right upper extremity or femoral pulses. Avoid assessment of pulses in the patient's neck or on the patient's left side. This minimizes confusion between the presence of an actual pulse and skeletal muscle contractions caused by the pacemaker.

- Once capture is achieved, continue pacing at an output level slightly higher (about 2 mA) than the threshold of initial electrical capture. For example, if capture is achieved at 90 mA, set the output level at 92 mA.

- Assess the patient's BP and level of responsiveness. Monitor the patient closely and record the ECG rhythm.

- Documentation should include the date and time pacing was initiated (including baseline and pacing rhythm strips), the current required to obtain capture, the pacing rate selected, the patient's responses to electrical and mechanical capture, medications administered during the procedure, and the date and time pacing was terminated.

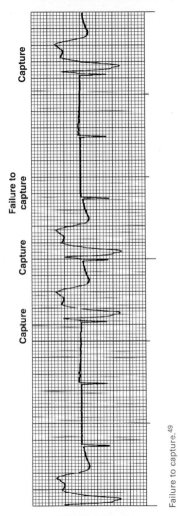

Failure to capture.[49]

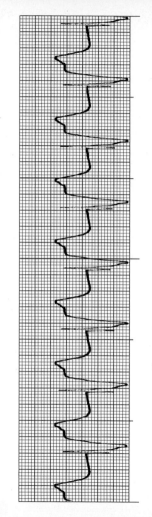

100% ventricular paced rhythm.[49]

IV THERAPY

IV cannulation is the placement of a catheter into a vein to gain access to the body's venous circulation. IV access may be achieved by cannulating a peripheral or central vein. During circulatory collapse or cardiac arrest, the preferred vascular access site is the largest, most accessible vein that does not require the interruption of resuscitation efforts. If no IV is in place before the arrest, establish IV access using a peripheral vein, preferably the antecubital or external jugular vein. During cardiac arrest, give IV drugs rapidly by bolus injection. Follow each drug with a 20-mL bolus of IV fluid and raise the extremity for 10 to 20 seconds to aid delivery of the drug(s) to the central circulation.

INDICATIONS

- Maintain hydration
- Restore fluid and electrolyte balance
- Provide fluids for resuscitation
- Administer medications, blood and blood components, nutrient solutions
- Obtain venous blood specimens for laboratory analysis

IV/Meds

PERIPHERAL VENOUS ACCESS

Advantages

- Effective route for medications during CPR
- Does not require interruption of CPR
- Easier to learn than central venous access
- Easily compressible site to reduce bleeding if an IV attempt is unsuccessful
- Results in fewer complications than central venous access

Disadvantages

- In circulatory collapse the vein may be difficult to access.
- Phlebitis is common with saphenous vein use.
- Should be used only for administration of isotonic solutions; hypertonic or irritating solutions may cause pain and phlebitis.
- In cardiac arrest, drugs given from a peripheral vein require 1 to 2 minutes to reach the central circulation.

CENTRAL VENOUS ACCESS

To access the central circulation, a central venous catheter (also called a *central line*) is inserted into the vena cava from the subclavian, jugular, or femoral vein. If peripheral IV access is unsuccessful during cardiac arrest, consider an intraosseous infusion before placing a central line.

Indications

- Emergency access to venous circulation when peripheral sites are not readily available
- Need for long-term IV therapy
- Administration of large volume of fluid
- Administration of hypertonic solutions,

caustic medications, or parenteral feeding solutions

- Placement of transvenous pacemaker electrodes
- Placement of central venous pressure or right heart catheters

Advantages

- Peak medication concentrations are higher and circulation times shorter when medications are administered via a central route compared with peripheral sites.

Disadvantages

- Special equipment (syringe, catheter, needle) required
- Excessive time (5-10 minutes) for placement
- High complication rate
- Skill deterioration (frequent practice required to maintain proficiency)
- Inability to initiate procedure while other patient care activities in progress

▆▆▆ INTRAOSSEOUS INFUSION ▆▆▆

When IV cannulation is unsuccessful or is taking too long, an intraosseous (IO) infusion is an alternative method of gaining access to the vascular system. An IO infusion is the process of infusing medications, fluids, and blood products into the bone marrow cavity for subsequent delivery to the venous circulation. Any medication or fluid that can be administered IV can be administered IO.

INDICATIONS

- Emergency administration of fluids and/or medications, especially in the setting of circulatory collapse where rapid vascular access is essential

- Difficult, delayed, or impossible IV access
- Burns or other injuries preventing venous access at other sites

TRACHEAL DRUG ADMINISTRATION

If IV or IO access cannot be achieved to give drugs during a cardiac arrest, the tracheal route can be used to give selected medications.

Studies have shown that naloxone, atropine, vasopressin, epinephrine, and lidocaine are medications that are absorbed via the trachea. The tracheal route of drug administration is not preferred because multiple studies have shown that giving resuscitation drugs tracheally results in lower blood concentrations than the same dose given IV.

The recommended dose of some drugs that can be given via the tracheal route is generally 2 to 2.5 times the IV dose, although the optimum tracheal dose of most drugs is unknown.

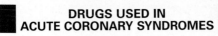

DRUGS USED IN
ACUTE CORONARY SYNDROMES

Oxygen	
Mechanism of Action	• Increases oxygen tension • Increases hemoglobin saturation if ventilation is supported • Improves tissue oxygenation when circulation is maintained
Indications	• Cardiac or respiratory arrest • Suspected hypoxemia of any cause • Any suspected cardiopulmonary emergency, especially complaints of shortness of breath and/or suspected ischemic chest pain
Dosing	Spontaneously breathing patient—best guided by pulse oximetry*, blood gases, and patient tolerance to oxygen delivery device. • Nasal cannula (0.25 to 8 L/min) • Simple face mask (5 to 10 L/min) • Partial rebreather mask (6 to 10 L/min) • Nonrebreather mask (10 L/min) Cardiac arrest—positive-pressure ventilation with 100% oxygen
Precautions	Toxicity possible with prolonged administration of high flow oxygen

*Pulse oximetry is inaccurate in low cardiac output states or with vasoconstriction.

Nitroglycerin	
Mechanism of Action	• Relaxes vascular smooth muscle; including dilation of the coronary arteries (particularly in the area of plaque disruption), the peripheral arterial bed, and venous capacitance vessels • Dilation of postcapillary vessels → peripheral pooling of blood → decreases venous return to the heart → decreases preload • Arteriolar relaxation reduces systemic vascular resistance and arterial pressure (afterload)
Indications	Sublingual tablets or spray: • Ongoing ischemic chest discomfort
Dosing (Adult)	Sublingual or spray • Give a nitroglycerin tablet (or spray) every 5 minutes up to 3 doses if the patient's SBP remains > 90 mm Hg or no more than 30 mm Hg below baseline and the heart rate remains between 50 and 100 bpm*

LV, Left ventricular.

O'Connor RE, Brady W, Brooks SC, et al. Part 10: acute coronary syndromes: 2010 American Heart Association Guidelines for Cardiopulmonary Resuscitation and Emergency Cardiovascular Care. *Circulation.* 2010;122 (suppl 3):S787–S817.

Nitroglycerin—cont'd

Precautions	Primary side effect is hypotension. Other side effects include tachycardia, bradycardia, headache, palpitations, syncope
Contraindications	• Use of a phosphodiesterase inhibitor such as sildenafil (Viagra) within 24 hours or tadalafil (Cialis) within 48 hours before NTG administration • Suspected inferior wall MI with possible right ventricular MI • Hypotension (SBP < 90 mm Hg or < 30 mm Hg below baseline) • Extreme bradycardia (<50 bpm) • Tachycardia (>100 bpm) in the absence of heart failure • Uncorrected hypovolemia • Inadequate cerebral circulation
Special Considerations	• Hypotension may worsen myocardial ischemia. Hypotension usually responds to administration of IV fluids. **Establishing an IV before giving SL nitroglycerin is strongly recommended.** • Significant hypotension may occur in the presence of right ventricular infarction.

SBP, Systolic blood pressure; *SL,* sublingual; *IV,* intravenous; *MI,* myocardial infarction.

Morphine Sulfate

Mechanism of Action	• Reduces pain of ischemia • Reduces anxiety • Increases venous capacitance (venous pooling) and decreases venous return (preload) • Decreases systemic vascular resistance (afterload) • Decreases myocardial oxygen demand
Indications	Unstable angina (UA)/non-ST-elevation MI (NSTEMI): Reasonable for patients whose symptoms are not relieved despite NTG or whose symptoms recur despite adequate anti-ischemic therapy* ST-elevation MI (STEMI): Analgesic of choice for patients with STEMI who experience persistent chest discomfort unresponsive to nitrates†
Dosing (Adult)	UA/NSTEMI: 1 to 5 mg IV STEMI: 2 to 4 mg IV with increments of 2 to 8 mg IV repeated at 5- to 15-min intervals
Precautions	Watch closely for: • Bradycardia • CNS depression • Nausea/vomiting • Respiratory depression • Hypotension
Contraindications	• Hypersensitivity to morphine/opiates • Respiratory depression • CNS depression due to head injury, overdose, poisoning, etc. • Increased intracranial pressure • Asthma (relative) • Undiagnosed abdominal pain • Hypovolemia • Hypotension
Special Considerations	Ensure a narcotic antagonist and airway equipment is within reach before giving

* and †: For reference see next page.

Naloxone

Mechanism of Action	While the mechanism of action of naloxone is not fully understood, evidence suggests naloxone antagonizes the effects of opiates by competing for the same receptor sites, thereby preventing or reversing the effects of narcotics including respiratory depression, sedation, and hypotension.
Indications	• Complete or partial reversal of narcotic depression, including respiratory depression, induced by opioids including natural and synthetic narcotics, propoxyphene, methadone and the narcotic-antagonist analgesics: nalbuphine, pentazocine and butorphanol. • Diagnosis of suspected acute opioid overdosage
Dosing (Adult)	IV, IM, SubQ—known or suspected narcotic overdose Initial dose 0.4 mg to 2 mg. If the desired degree of counteraction and improvement in respiratory function is not obtained, it may be repeated at 2 to 3 minute intervals.* If no response is observed after 10 mg of naloxone have been given, reevaluate diagnosis. IM or SubQ administration may be necessary if IV route is not available.

Continued.

IV, Intravenous; IM, intramuscular; SubQ, subcutaneous.

Mosby's Drug Consult, St Louis, 2006, Mosby.

Morphine Sulfate: *Anderson JL, Adams CD, Antman EM, et al. ACC/AHA 2007 guidelines for the management of patients with unstable angina/non–ST-elevation myocardial infarction: a report of the American College of Cardiology/American Heart Association Task Force on Practice Guidelines (Writing Committee to Revise the 2002 Guidelines for the Management of Patients With Unstable Angina/Non–ST-Elevation Myocardial Infarction): developed in collaboration with the American College of Emergency Physicians, American College of Physicians, Society for Academic Emergency Medicine, Society for Cardiovascular Angiography and Interventions, and Society of Thoracic Surgeons, J Am Coll Cardiol 50: e1–e157, 2007.

†O'Connor RE, Brady W, Brooks SC, et al. Part 10: acute coronary syndromes: 2010 American Heart Association Guidelines for Cardiopulmonary Resuscitation and Emergency Cardiovascular Care. Circulation. 2010;122(suppl 3):S787–S817.

Naloxone—cont'd	
Precautions	Abrupt reversal of narcotic depression may result in nausea, vomiting, sweating, tachycardia, increased blood pressure, tremulousness, seizures, cardiac arrest
Contraindications	Known hypersensitivity to the medication
Special Considerations	• Ineffective if respiratory depression due to hypnotics, sedatives, anesthetics, or other nonnarcotic CNS depressants • Effects of narcotics are usually longer than those of naloxone thus, respiratory depression may return when naloxone has worn off. Monitor the patient closely. • Naloxone can also be given by the intranasal or endotracheal routes. The IV, IM, or SubQ routes are preferred over the tracheal route.†

CNS, Central nervous system.

†2005 American Heart Association guidelines for cardiopulmonary resuscitation and emergency cardiovascular care, part 10.2, toxicology in ECC, *Circulation* 112(suppl IV):IV-129, 2005.

Aspirin

Mechanism of Action	Blocks synthesis of thromboxane A_2, inhibiting platelet aggregation.
Indications	• Chest discomfort or other signs/symptoms suggestive of an acute coronary syndrome (unless hypersensitive to aspirin) • ECG changes suggestive of acute MI
Dosing (Adult)	162 to 325 mg ,chewed, if no history of aspirin allergy or signs of active or recent gastrointestinal bleeding*
Precautions	• Asthma (relative contraindication) • Active ulcer disease (relative contraindication)
Contraindications	• Hypersensitivity to aspirin and/or non-steroidal anti-inflammatory agents • Recent history of GI bleeding • Bleeding disorders (hemophilia)
Special Considerations	• Use with caution in the patient with a history of asthma, nasal polyps, or nasal allergies. Anaphylactic reactions in sensitive patients have occurred. • Consider ticlopidine, or clopidogrel if aspirin allergy, intolerant, or ineffective • Rectal suppository may be used for patients who cannot take aspirin orally

*O'Connor RE, Brady W, Brooke SC, et al, Part 10: acute coronary syndromes: 2010 American Heart Association Guidelines for Cardiopulmonary Resuscitation and Emergency Cardiovascular Care, *Circulation.* 2010;122 (suppl 3):S787–S817.

Fibrinolytics

Mechanism of Action	Fibrinolytics work by altering plasmin in the body, which then breaks down fibrinogen and fibrin clots
Indications	• Improvement of ventricular function following ST-elevation MI (STEMI) with onset of symptoms of ≤ 12 hours and ECG findings consistent with STEMI • tPA may be used in acute ischemic stroke, after intracranial hemorrhage has been excluded by CT scan or other diagnostic imaging • Acute pulmonary thromboembolism
Special Considerations	• Pay careful attention to all potential bleeding sites (including catheter insertion sites, arterial and venous puncture sites, cutdown sites, and needle puncture sites). • Some fibrinolytics are associated with an increased risk of bleeding or hemorrhage if used with heparin, oral anticoagulants, vitamin K antagonists, aspirin, or dipyridamole

Contraindications and Cautions for Fibrinolytic Use in STEMI*

Absolute Contraindications	• Any prior intracranial hemorrhage • Known structural cerebrovascular lesion (e.g., AVM) • Known malignant intracranial neoplasm (primary or metastatic) • Ischemic stroke within 3 months EXCEPT acute ischemic stroke within 3 hours • Suspected aortic dissection • Active bleeding or bleeding diathesis (excluding menses) • Significant closed head trauma or facial trauma within 3 months
Cautions and Relative Contraindications	1. History of chronic, severe, poorly controlled hypertension 2. Severe uncontrolled hypertension on presentation (SBP > 180 mm Hg or DBP > 110 mm Hg) (could be an absolute contraindication in low-risk patients with myocardial infarction) 3. History of prior ischemic stroke within 3 months, dementia, or intracranial pathology not contraindicated 4. Traumatic or prolonged (10 minutes) CPR or major surgery (<3 weeks) 5. Internal bleeding (within 2-4 weeks) 6. Noncompressible vascular punctures 7. For streptokinase/anistreplase: prior exposure (5 days ago) or allergic reaction 8. Pregnancy 9. Active peptic ulcer 10. Current anticoagulant use: higher INR means higher risk of bleeding

AVM, Arteriovenous malformation; *SBP*, systolic blood pressure; *DBP*, diastolic blood pressure; *CPR*, cardiopulmonary resuscitation; *INR*, international normalized ratio.

From Antman EM et al:
www.acc.org/clinical/guidelines/stemi/index.pdf/.
Accessed 2004.

*Viewed as advisory for clinical decision making and may not be all-inclusive or definitive.

DRUGS USED FOR CONTROL OF HEART RHYTHM AND RATE

Adenosine

Mechanism of Action	• Found naturally in all body cells • Rapidly metabolized in the blood vessels • Slows sinus rate • Slows conduction time through AV node • Can interrupt reentry pathways through AV node • Can restore sinus rhythm in reentry SVT, including SVT associated with Wolff-Parkinson-White Syndrome
Indications*	• Stable narrow-QRS regular tachycardias • Unstable narrow-QRS regular tachycardia while preparations are made for synchronized cardioversion • Stable, regular, wide-QRS tachycardia
Dosing (Adult)*	• 6 mg rapid IV push over 1-3 seconds. Decrease the dose to 3 mg in patients on dipyridamole (Persantine), carbamazepine (Tegretol), those with transplanted hearts, or if given via a central IV line. Consider increasing the dose in patients on theophylline, caffeine, or theobromine. • If no response within 1-2 minutes, give 12 mg. May repeat 12 mg dose once in 1-2 minutes.

*Neumar RW, Otto CW, Link MS, et al. Part 8: Adult advanced cardiovascular life support: 2010 American Heart Association Guidelines for Cardiopulmonary Resuscitation and Emergency Cardiovascular Care. *Circulation.* 2010;122(suppl 3):S729 –S767.

Adenosine—cont'd	
Precautions	Side effects common but transient and usually resolve within 1-2 minutes • Cardiovascular: Facial flushing (common), chest pain (common), headache, sweating, palpitations, hypotension • Respiratory: Shortness of breath/dyspnea (common), chest pressure, hyperventilation • Central nervous system: Lightheadedness, dizziness, tingling in arms, numbness, apprehension, blurred vision, burning sensation, heaviness in arms, neck and back pain • Gastrointestinal: Nausea, metallic taste, tightness in throat, pressure in groin Use with caution with obstructive lung disease not associated with bronchoconstriction (emphysema, bronchitis)
Contraindications	• Poison/drug-induced tachycardia • Bronchoconstriction or bronchospasm (asthma) • Second- or third-degree AV block • Sick sinus syndrome (except in patients with a functioning artificial pacemaker)
Special Considerations	• Recommended IV site is the antecubital fossa. Follow each dose immediately with a 20-mL normal saline flush and raise the arm for 10-20 seconds. Use the injection port nearest the hub of the IV catheter. **Constant ECG monitoring is essential.** • Must be injected into the IV tubing as fast as possible (over a period of seconds). Failure may result in medication breakdown while still in the IV tubing. • Discontinue in any patient who develops severe respiratory difficulty

Amiodarone

Mechanism of Action	• Slows conduction in the His-Purkinje system and in accessory pathway of patients with Wolff-Parkinson-White syndrome • Inhibits alpha- and beta-receptors and possesses both vagolytic and calcium-channel blocking properties • Lengthens action potential duration and increases refractory period in all cardiac tissues including the SA node, AV node, atrial cells, Purkinje fibers, and in the ventricular myocardium
Indications	• Pulseless VT/VF (after CPR, defibrillation, and a vasopressor) • Stable narrow-QRS tachycardias if the rhythm persists despite vagal maneuvers or adenosine or the tachycardia is recurrent • To control ventricular rate in atrial fibrillation • To control ventricular rate in pre-excited atrial dysrhythmias with conduction over an accessory pathway • Stable monomorphic VT • Polymorphic VT with normal QT interval
Dosing (Adult)	**Cardiac arrest–Pulseless VT/VF** • Initial bolus–300 mg IV/IO bolus.* **Other indications:** • Loading dose–150 mg IV bolus over 10 minutes (15 mg/min). May repeat every 10 min as needed. After conversion, follow with a 1 mg/min infusion for 6 hours and then a 0.5 mg/min maintenance infusion over 18 hours.‡ • Maximum cumulative dose 2.2 g IV/24 hours.

*Neumar RW, Otto CW, Link MS, et al. Part 8: Adult advanced cardiovascular life support: 2010 American Heart Association Guidelines for Cardiopulmonary Resuscitation and Emergency Cardiovascular Care. *Circulation.* 2010;122(suppl 3):S729 –S767.

Amiodarone—cont'd	
Precautions	• Hypotension and bradycardia are most common side effects. Slow infusion rate or discontinue if seen.
Contraindications	• Known hypersensitivity • Severe sinus-node dysfunction causing marked sinus bradycardia • Second- and third-degree AV block • Syncope due to bradycardia (except when used with a pacemaker) • Use with caution in patients with uncorrected electrolyte abnormalities, particularly hypokalemia and/or hypomagnesemia, because these conditions may predispose the patient to proarrhythmias
Special Considerations	• Additive effect with other medications that prolong the QT interval (e.g., Class Ia antiarrhythmics, phenothiazines, tricyclic antidepressants, thiazide diuretics, sotalol) • In therapeutic doses, amiodarone has only a mild negative effect on myocardial contractility. This is the reason it appears in multiple algorithms involving patients experiencing dysrhythmias but who have signs of heart failure.

‡Neumar RW, Otto CW, Link MS, et al. Part 8: Adult advanced cardiovascular life support: 2010 American Heart Association Guidelines for Cardiopulmonary Resuscitation and Emergency Cardiovascular Care. *Circulation.* 2010;122(suppl 3):S729 –S767.

Atropine

Mechanism of Action	**Cardiovascular** • Increases heart rate (positive chronotropic effect) by accelerating SA node discharge rate and blocking vagus nerve • Increases conduction velocity (positive dromotropic effect) • Little or no effect on force of contraction (inotropic effect) • **May** restore cardiac rhythm in asystole or slow pulseless electrical activity (PEA) **Respiratory** – Relaxes bronchial smooth muscle (bronchodilation); decreases body secretions (lungs, bronchi, GI tract, sweat, saliva) **GI/GU** – Decreased GI motility and secretions, urinary retention **Other** – Pupil dilation, decreased sweat production
Indications	• First-line drug for symptomatic narrow-QRS bradycardia
Dosing (Adult)	• 0.5 mg IV push every 3 to 5 min to a total dose of 3 mg*
Precautions	• Do not push slowly or in smaller than recommended doses. Small doses (under 0.5 mg) produce modest paradoxical cardiac slowing that may last two minutes. • May result in tachycardia, palpitations, and ventricular ectopy. • Use with caution in acute MI. Excessive increases in heart rate may further worsen ischemia or increase size of infarction

*Neumar RW, Otto CW, Link MS, et al. Part 8: Adult advanced cardiovascular life support: 2010 American Heart Association Guidelines for Cardiopulmonary Resuscitation and Emergency Cardiovascular Care. *Circulation.* 2010;122(suppl 3):S729 –S767.

Beta-blockers

Mechanism of Action	• Slow sinus rate • Depress AV conduction • Reduce blood pressure • Decrease myocardial oxygen consumption
Indications*	Stable narrow-QRS tachycardias if the rhythm persists despite vagal maneuvers or adenosine or the tachycardia is recurrent For ventricular rate control in atrial fibrillation and atrial flutter if no signs of heart failure Specific forms of polymorphic ventricular tachycardia
Precautions	• Some beta-blockers should be used with caution in patients with impaired renal or liver function
Contraindications	• Signs of heart failure • Evidence of a low output state (such as oliguria) • Increased risk for cardiogenic shock • PR interval greater than 0.24 seconds (relative) • Second- or third-degree heart block (relative) • Active asthma (relative) • Reactive airway disease (relative)
Special Considerations	• Use with caution in conjunction with medications that slow conduction (e.g., digitalis, calcium channel blockers) and in those that decrease myocardial contractility (e.g., calcium channel blockers). • IV administration may be warranted at the time of presentation to patients who have severe hypertension or tachydysrhythmias in the setting of acute coronary syndromes and who do not have contraindications to beta blockade.

*Neumar RW, Otto CW, Link MS, et al. Part 8: adult advanced cardiovascular life support: 2010 American Heart Association Guidelines for Cardiopulmonary Resuscitation and Emergency Cardiovascular Care. *Circulation.* 2010;122(suppl 3):S729 –S767.

Digitalis

Mechanism of Action	• Slows conduction through AV node (prolonging PR interval) • In atrial flutter or fibrillation, decreases number of atrial impulses reaching the ventricles, thus decreasing the ventricular response (- chronotropic effect) • Increases force and velocity of myocardial contraction (+ inotropic effect) • Increases cardiac output
Indications	*Limited use in emergency cardiac care*
Precautions	• Toxic-to-therapeutic ratio is narrow • May result in toxicity in patients with hypokalemia or hypomagnesemia because potassium or magnesium depletion sensitizes the myocardium to digoxin • Hypercalcemia predisposes the patient to digitalis toxicity • May cause severe sinus bradycardia or SA block in patients with pre-existing sinus node disease • May cause complete AV block in patients with pre-existing incomplete AV block.
Contraindications	• Known hypersensitivity • Digitalis toxicity
Special Considerations	• ACE inhibitors have largely replaced digoxin as first-line therapy for CHF due to systolic dysfunction. • In patients with atrial fibrillation or atrial flutter, IV calcium-channel blockers or beta-blockers are generally more effective than digoxin for initial control of ventricular rate.

Diltiazem	
Mechanism of Action*	Inhibits movement of calcium ions across cell membranes in the heart and vascular smooth muscle, resulting in: • Relaxation of coronary vascular smooth muscle • Dilation of both large and small coronary arteries • Decreased sinoatrial and atrioventricular conduction • Decreased myocardial oxygen demand Produces antihypertensive effects primarily by relaxation of vascular smooth muscle and a resultant decrease in peripheral vascular resistance
Indications†	• Stable narrow-QRS tachycardia if the rhythm persists despite vagal maneuvers or adenosine or the tachycardia is recurrent • To control the ventricular rate in patients with atrial fibrillation or atrial flutter
Dosing (Adult)†	Initial dose 0.25 mg/kg IV bolus over 2 min. If needed, follow in 15 min with 0.35 mg/kg over 2 min. Subsequent IV bolus doses should be individualized for each patient.

Continued.

* *Mosby's Drug Consult,* St Louis, 2006 Mosby.

†Neumar RW, Otto CW, Link MS, et al. Part 8: Adult advanced cardiovascular life support: 2010 American Heart Association Guidelines for Cardiopulmonary Resuscitation and Emergency Cardiovascular Care. *Circulation.* 2010,122(suppl 3):S729 –S767

Diltiazem—cont'd

Precautions	• Avoid calcium channel blockers in patients with wide-QRS tachycardia unless it is known with certainty to be supraventricular in origin. (may precipitate VF) • Avoid in patients with heart failure and atrial fibrillation or atrial flutter associated with known preexcitation (e.g., Wolff-Parkinson-White [WPW]) syndrome.
Contraindications	• Wide-QRS tachycardia of uncertain origin • Poison/drug-induced tachycardias • Digitalis toxicity (may worsen heart block) • Atrial fibrillation or atrial flutter with an accessory bypass tract (WPW) • Sick-sinus syndrome (bradycardia-tachycardia syndrome) except with a functioning ventricular pacemaker • Severe CHF • Second or third-degree AV block • Hypotension (SBP <90 mm Hg) • Cardiogenic shock
Special Considerations	• Concurrent use of amiodarone and diltiazem can result in bradycardia and decreased cardiac output by an unknown mechanism • Monitor closely for hypotension and AV block. • IV calcium channel blockers and IV beta-blockers should not be given together or in close proximity (within a few hours) – may cause severe hypotension

Epinephrine

Mechanism of Action	Stimulates alpha, beta$_1$, and beta$_2$ receptors • Alpha-agonist – constricts arterioles in skin, mucosa, kidneys, and viscera → increased systemic vascular resistance • Beta$_1$ agonist – increases force of contraction (+ inotropic effect), increases heart rate (+ chronotropic effect) → increased myocardial workload and oxygen requirements • Beta$_2$ agonist – relaxation of bronchial smooth muscle, dilation of vessels in skeletal muscle; dilation of cerebral, pulmonary, coronary, and hepatic vessels
Indications	• Cardiac arrest – VF, pulseless VT, asystole, pulseless electrical activity (PEA) • Symptomatic bradycardia
Dosing (Adult)	**Cardiac Arrest** • IV/IO: 1 mg (10-mL) of 1:10,000 solution, follow with 20-mL fluid flush. May repeat 1 mg dose every 3 to 5 minutes • Tracheal: 2 to 2.5 mg diluted in 5 to 10 mL of sterile water or normal saline **Symptomatic Bradycardia or Hypotension*** • Continuous infusion at 2 to 10 mcg/min
Precautions	Increases myocardial oxygen demand
Special Considerations	Should not be administered in the same IV line as alkaline solutions – inactivates epinephrine.

*Neumar RW, Otto CW, Link MS, et al. Part 8: Adult advanced cardiovascular life support: 2010 American Heart Association Guidelines for Cardiopulmonary Resuscitation and Emergency Cardiovascular Care. *Circulation.* 2010;122(suppl 3):S729 –S767.

Lidocaine hydrochloride

Mechanism of Action	Decreases conduction in ischemic cardiac tissue without adversely affecting normal conduction
Indications	• Stable monomorphic VT • Pulseless VT/VF that persists after defibrillation and vasopressor administration (if amiodarone is not available)
Dosing (Adult)	• Initial dose: 1 to 1.5 mg/kg IV/IO bolus. Consider repeat dose (0.5 to 0.75 mg/kg) in 5 to 10 minutes. Cumulative IV/IO bolus dose should not exceed 3 mg/kg • Maintenance infusion: 1 to 4 mg/min. • Tracheal dose: 2 to 3 mg/kg
Precautions	Signs and symptoms of lidocaine toxicity are primarily CNS related – dizziness, drowsiness, mild agitation, tinnitus, slurred speech, hearing impairment, disorientation and confusion, muscle twitching, seizures, and respiratory arrest.
Contraindications	• Hypersensitivity to lidocaine or amide-type local anesthetics • Severe degrees of sinoatrial, atrioventricular, or intraventricular block in the absence of an artificial pacemaker • Stokes-Adams syndrome (sudden recurring episodes of loss of consciousness caused by transient interruption of cardiac output by incomplete or complete heart block) • Wolff-Parkinson-White syndrome
Special Considerations	Lidocaine may be *lethal* in a bradycardia with a ventricular escape rhythm.

Magnesium sulfate

Mechanism of Action	• Essential for activity of many enzyme systems • Plays an important role with regard to neurochemical transmission and muscular excitability
Indications	Polymorphic VT with prolonged QT interval (Torsades de Pointes)
Dosing (Adult)*	If pulseless, give 1 to 2 g IV diluted in 10 mL D$_5$W. If pulse present, give 1 to 2 g IV diluted in 50 to 100 mL D$_5$W over 15 min.
Precautions	• Caution should be used in patients receiving digitalis • Use with caution in patients with impaired renal function • Use with caution in patients with preexisting heart blocks
Contraindications	• Respiratory depression • Hypocalcemia • Hypermagnesemia
Special Considerations	Signs and symptoms of magnesium overdose include: • Hypotension • Flushing, sweating • Bradycardia, AV block • Respiratory depression • Drowsiness, decreasing level of consciousness • Diminished reflexes or muscle weakness, flaccid paralysis Antidote = calcium

*Neumar RW, Otto CW, Link MS, et al. Part 8: Adult advanced cardiovascular life support: 2010 American Heart Association Guidelines for Cardiopulmonary Resuscitation and Emergency Cardiovascular Care. *Circulation.* 2010;122(suppl 3):S729–S767.

Procainamide

Mechanism of Action	• Prolongs the effective refractory period and action potential duration in the atria, ventricles, and His-Purkinje system • Suppresses ectopy in atrial and ventricular tissue • Prolongs the PR and QT intervals • Exerts a peripheral vasodilatory effect
Indications	• To control the ventricular rate in the patient with pre-excited atrial fibrillation • Stable monomorphic ventricular tachycardia
Dosing (Adult)*	20 to 50 mg/min IV infusion or 100 mg every 5 min until one of the following occurs: • Dysrhythmia resolves • Hypotension ensues • QRS prolongs by >50% of original width • Total dose of 17 mg/kg administered Maintenance infusion 1 to 4 mg/min.
Precautions	Use with caution with other medications that prolong the QT interval (e.g., phenothiazines, tricyclic antidepressants, thiazide diuretics, sotalol) During administration, carefully monitor the patient's ECG and blood pressure. If the blood pressure falls 15 mm Hg or more, procainamide administration should be temporarily discontinued. Watch the ECG closely for increasing PR and QT intervals, widening of the QRS complex, heart block, and/or onset of TdP. Reduce maintenance infusion rate in liver dysfunction, renal failure

*Neumar RW, Otto CW, Link MS, et al. Part 8: Adult advanced cardiovascular life support: 2010 American Heart Association Guidelines for Cardiopulmonary Resuscitation and Emergency Cardiovascular Care. *Circulation.* 2010;122(suppl 3):S729 –S767.

Procainamide—cont'd	
Contraindications	• Complete AV block in the absence of an artificial pacemaker • Patients sensitive to procaine or other ester-type local anesthetics • Lupus erythematosus • Patients with a prolonged QRS duration or QT interval because of the potential for heart block • Preexisting QT prolongation/Torsades de Pointes • Digitalis toxicity (procainamide may further depress conduction)

Sotalol	
Mechanism of Action	Sotalol is a Class III antiarrhythmic with non-selective beta-blockade activity. • Slows heart rate • Decreases AV nodal conduction • Increases AV nodal refractoriness • Prolongs the effective refractory period of atrial muscle, ventricular muscle, and AV accessory pathways (where present) in both anterograde and retrograde directions • Increases force of contraction
Indications*	• Stable monomorphic VT
Dosing (Adult)	1.5 mg/kg IV is the dose used in clinical studies U.S. packaging label recommends that any dose should be infused slowly over 5 hours
Precautions	• Because of its effect on cardiac repolarization (QT interval prolongation), TdP is the most common dysrhythmia associated with sotalol administration. The risk of TdP progressively increases with prolongation of the QT interval, and is worsened by reduction in heart rate and reduction in serum potassium. Patients with sustained VT and a history of CHF appear to have the highest risk for serious proarrhythmia • Should not be used in patients with hypokalemia or hypomagnesemia (these conditions can exaggerate the degree of QT prolongation, and increase the potential for TdP) • Bradycardia • Hypotension

*Neumar RW, Otto CW, Link MS, et al. Part 8: Adult advanced cardiovascular life support: 2010 American Heart Association Guidelines for Cardiopulmonary Resuscitation and Emergency Cardiovascular Care. *Circulation.* 2010;122(suppl 3):S729 –S767.

Sotalol—cont'd	
Contraindications	• Bronchial asthma • Sinus bradycardia • Second and third-degree AV block (unless a functioning pacemaker is present) • Congenital or acquired long QT syndromes • Cardiogenic shock • Uncontrolled CHF • Previous evidence of hypersensitivity to sotalol

Verapamil	
Mechanism of Action	Inhibits movement of calcium ions across cell membranes in the heart and vascular smooth muscle, resulting in: • Relaxation of coronary vascular smooth muscle • Dilation of both large and small coronary arteries • Decreased sinoatrial and atrioventricular conduction • Decreased myocardial oxygen demand
Indications*	• Stable narrow-QRS tachycardia if the rhythm persists despite vagal maneuvers or adenosine or the tachycardia is recurrent • To control the ventricular rate in patients with atrial fibrillation or atrial flutter
Dosing (Adult)*	2.5- to 5-mg slow IV push over 2 minutes (give over 3 to 4 min in older adults or when BP is within the lower range of normal). May repeat with 5 to 10 mg in 15 to 30 min (if no response and BP remains normal or elevated). Maximum total dose 20 to 30 mg.

*Neumar RW, Otto CW, Link MS, et al. Part 8: Adult advanced cardiovascular life support: 2010 American Heart Association Guidelines for Cardiopulmonary Resuscitation and Emergency Cardiovascular Care. *Circulation*. 2010;122(suppl 3):S729 –S767.

Verapamil—cont'd

Precautions	• Avoid calcium channel blockers in patients with wide-QRS tachycardia unless it is known with certainty to be supraventricular in origin. (may precipitate VF) • Calcium channel blockers decrease peripheral resistance and can worsen hypotension. Monitor BP, heart rate, and ECG closely. • IV calcium channel blockers and IV beta-blockers should not be given together or in close proximity (within a few hours)—may cause severe hypotension
Contraindications	• Wide-QRS tachycardia of uncertain origin • Poison/drug-induced tachycardias • Digitalis toxicity (may worsen heart block) • Atrial fibrillation or atrial flutter with an accessory bypass tract (WPW) • Sick-sinus syndrome (bradycardia-tachycardia syndrome) except with a functioning ventricular pacemaker • Severe CHF • Second or third-degree AV block • Hypotension (systolic BP less than 90 mm Hg) • Cardiogenic shock
Special Considerations	During administration, monitor closely for hypotension and AV block.

DRUGS USED TO IMPROVE CARDIAC OUTPUT AND BLOOD PRESSURE

Calcium Chloride	
Mechanism of Action	• Fifth most abundant element in the body • Essential for functional integrity of nervous and muscular systems • Necessary for normal cardiac contractility and coagulation of blood • Increases force of cardiac contraction (positive inotropic effect) • Antidote for magnesium sulfate
Indications	• Known or suspected acute hyperkalemia • Hypocalcemia • Calcium channel blocker toxicity/overdose • Pretreatment for calcium channel blocker administration • Magnesium toxicity
Dosing (Adult)	Hyperkalemia: 500 to 1000 mg (5 to 10 mL) IV of a 10% solution (100 mg/mL) over 2 to 5 minutes.* Dosage should be titrated by constant monitoring of ECG changes during administration.

*Vanden Hoek TL, Morrison LJ, Shuster M, et al. Part 12: Cardiac arrest in special situations: 2010 American Heart Association guidelines for cardiopulmonary resuscitation and emergency cardiovascular care. *Circulation.* 2010;122(suppl 3):S829 –S861.

Calcium Chloride—cont'd	
Precautions	• Do not give calcium intramuscularly or subcutaneously—can cause severe tissue necrosis, sloughing, or abscess formation.
	• Irritating to veins. Monitor IV site closely. Ensure patency of IV line before giving. Patient may experience pain, burning at the IV site, severe venous thrombosis, and severe tissue necrosis if solution extravasates. Patient may complain of "heat waves," tingling, and/or a metallic taste if given too rapidly.
	• Calcium chloride administration may be accompanied by peripheral vasodilation, with a moderate fall in blood pressure.
	• Use with caution in patients taking digitalis—increases ventricular irritability and can precipitate digitalis toxicity
Contraindications	Hypercalcemia, concurrent digitalis therapy (relative contraindication), kidney stones, VF
Special Considerations	• Incompatible with all medications. Flush line before and after giving.
	• Concurrent administration of sodium bicarbonate and calcium chloride will produce a precipitate, calcium carbonate (chalk).

Dobutamine

Mechanism of Action	• Stimulates alpha, beta$_1$, and beta$_2$ receptors • Potent inotropic effect (i.e., increased myocardial contractility, increased stroke volume, increased cardiac output) • Less chronotropic effect (heart rate) • Minimal alpha effect (vasoconstriction)
Indications	• Short-term management of patients with cardiac decompensation due to depressed contractility (CHF, pulmonary congestion)
Dosing (Adult)	• Continuous IV infusion. Usual dose is 2 to 20 mcg/kg/min IV, but patient response varies.
Precautions	• Tachycardia may occur with high doses, although this occurs less commonly than with dopamine. • Continuously monitor ECG and blood pressure
Contraindications	• Hypersensitivity to sulfites or dobutamine • Tachydysrhythmias • Severe hypotension • Hypertrophic aortic stenosis
Special Considerations	• May cause a marked increase in heart rate or blood pressure, especially systolic pressure • Correct hypovolemia before treatment with dobutamine • Use with tricyclic antidepressants can cause an increased adrenergic effect and possibly result in severe hypertensive crisis or cardiac dysrhythmias

Dopamine

Mechanism of Action	• Naturally occurring immediate precursor of norepinephrine in the body • Pharmacologic effects change with increasing dosage • Stimulates dopaminergic, beta, and alpha-adrenergic receptor sites
Indications	• Temporizing measure in the management of symptomatic bradycardia that has not responded to atropine, or for which atropine is inappropriate, while awaiting availability of a pacemaker • Hypotension that occurs after return of spontaneous circulation • Hemodynamically significant hypotension in the absence of hypovolemia
Dosing (Adult)*	• Dopamine is given as a continuous IV infusion of 2 to 10 mcg/kg/min. • Increase infusion rate according to BP and other clinical responses.
Precautions	• Correct hypovolemia before beginning dopamine therapy for the treatment of hypotension and shock.
Contraindications	• Hypersensitivity to sulfites or dopamine • Hypovolemia • Pheochromocytoma • Uncorrected tachydysrhythmias or VF • MAO inhibitors
Special Considerations	• Extravasation into surrounding tissue may cause necrosis and sloughing • Gradually taper drug before discontinuing the infusion. Monitor blood pressure, ECG, and drip rate closely. • Dilute before giving (or used premixed bag of IV solution). Do not give as an IV bolus. Only infuse via infusion pump.

*Neumar RW, Otto CW, Link MS, et al. Part 8: Adult advanced cardiovascular life support: 2010 American Heart Association Guidelines for Cardiopulmonary Resuscitation and Emergency Cardiovascular Care. *Circulation.* 2010;122(suppl 3):S729 –S767.

Norepinephrine

Mechanism of Action	• Norepinephrine functions as a peripheral vasoconstrictor (alpha-adrenergic action) and as an inotropic stimulator of the heart and dilator of coronary arteries (beta-adrenergic action) • Alpha activity dominant • Increases myocardial oxygen demand
Indications	• Cardiogenic shock • Severe hypotension (systolic BP <70 mm Hg) not due to hypovolemia
Dosing (Adult)*	• 0.5 to 1 mcg/min by continuous IV infusion titrated to improve blood pressure (up to 30 mcg/min); usual dose range is 8 to 12 mcg/min • When discontinuing infusion, taper off gradually
Precautions	• Use with extreme caution in patients receiving monoamine oxidase inhibitors (MAOI) or antidepressants of the triptyline or imipramine types, because severe, prolonged hypertension may result
Contraindications	• Hypersensitivity to sulfites or norepinephrine • Hypotension due to hypovolemia (except in emergencies) • Mesenteric or peripheral vascular thrombosis • Halothane or cyclopropane anesthesia (possibility of fatal dysrhythmias) • Pregnancy (may cause fetal anoxia or hypoxia)

*2005 American Heart Association guidelines for cardiopulmonary resuscitation and emergency cardiovascular care, part 7.4, monitoring and medications, *Circulation* 112(suppl IV):IV-79, 2005.

Norepinephrine—cont'd

Special Considerations	• Should be administered via an infusion pump into a central vein or a large peripheral vein (e.g., antecubital vein) to reduce the risk of necrosis of the overlying skin from prolonged vasoconstriction.
	• Extravasation into surrounding tissue may cause necrosis and sloughing. Antidote for extravasation = phentolamine (Regitine).
	• Monitor blood pressure every 2 to 3 minutes until stabilized, then every 5 minutes. Monitor the patient's ECG continuously.

Vasopressin

Mechanism of Action	Causes constriction of peripheral, cerebral, pulmonary, and coronary vessels
Indications	Cardiac arrest
Dosing (Adult)*	One time dose of 40 units IV/IO push—May be used in place of first or second dose of epinephrine in cardiac arrest
Precautions	• Can increase peripheral vascular resistance and provoke cardiac ischemia and angina pectoris • Nausea and vomiting • Tremors • Tissue necrosis if extravasation occurs
Contraindications	• Hypersensitivity • Responsive patient with coronary artery disease or peripheral vascular disease
Special Considerations	• Half-life approximately 10 to 20 minutes

*Neumar RW, Otto CW, Link MS, et al. Part 8: Adult advanced cardiovascular life support: 2010 American Heart Association Guidelines for Cardiopulmonary Resuscitation and Emergency Cardiovascular Care. *Circulation.* 2010;122(suppl 3):S729 –S767.

VASODILATORS

Sodium Nitroprusside

Mechanism of Action	Direct-acting arterial and venous vasodilator • Relaxes vascular smooth muscle with consequent dilation of peripheral arteries and veins; other smooth muscle (e.g., uterus, duodenum) is not affected • Nitroprusside is more active on veins than on arteries • Venodilation promotes peripheral pooling of blood and decreases venous return to the heart, thereby reducing preload • Arteriolar relaxation reduces systemic vascular resistance (afterload) • Dilates coronary arteries
Indications	Immediate reduction of blood pressure in a hypertensive emergency or hypertensive urgency
Precautions	Nitroprusside can cause precipitous decreases in BP. In patients not properly monitored, these decreases can lead to irreversible ischemic injuries or death. Monitor for signs of cyanide toxicity. Solution is sensitive to certain wavelengths of light, and must be protected from light during clinical use
Contraindications	Hypotension, severe refractory CHF

Furosemide

Mechanism of Action	• Inhibits the reabsorption of sodium and chloride in the ascending limb of the loop of Henle, resulting in an increase in the urinary excretion of sodium, chloride, and water → profound diuresis • Venodilation — increases venous capacitance, decreases preload (venous return)
Indications	Adjunctive therapy in acute pulmonary edema (systolic BP >90 to 100 mm Hg without signs and symptoms of shock)
Dosing (Adult)*	The initial dose is 0.5 to 1 mg/kg IV push given at a rate no faster than 20 mg/minute.
Precautions	Ototoxicity and resulting transient deafness can occur with rapid administration. Do not exceed the recommended rate of administration. Furosemide should be administered cautiously in patients with: • Diabetes mellitus • Dehydration • Severe renal disease Patients with sulfonamide hypersensitivity or thiazide diuretic hypersensitivity may also be hypersensitive to furosemide.
Contraindications	• Hypersensitivity to furosemide or sulfonamides • Hypovolemia • Severe electrolyte depletion • Hypotension • Anuria
Special Considerations	Can cause excessive fluid loss and dehydration, resulting in hypovolemia and electrolyte imbalance

*2005 American Heart Association guidelines for cardiopulmonary resuscitation and emergency cardiovascular care, part 7.4, monitoring and medications, *Circulation* 112(suppl IV):IV-82, 2005.

Sodium Bicarbonate

Mechanism of Action	• Increases plasma bicarbonate • Buffers excess hydrogen ion concentration • Raises blood pH • Reverses clinical manifestations of acidosis
Indications	• Known preexisting hyperkalemia • Preexisting metabolic acidosis • Overdose – tricyclic antidepressants, procainamide
Dosing (Adult)	• Initial dose 1 mEq/kg IV bolus.* 1/2 the initial dose may be repeated every 10 minutes thereafter • Repeated IV boluses of 1 to 2 mEq/kg may be needed when sodium bicarbonate is used to treat drug-induced arrhythmias and hypotension.†
Precautions	Extravasation may lead to tissue inflammation and necrosis.
Contraindications	• Significant metabolic or respiratory alkalosis • Severe pulmonary edema

Continued.

*2005 American Heart Association guidelines for cardiopulmonary resuscitation and emergency cardiovascular care, part 7.4, monitoring and medications, *Circulation* 112(suppl IV):IV-82, 2005.

†2005 American Heart Association guidelines for cardiopulmonary resuscitation and emergency cardiovascular care, part 10.2, toxicology in emergency cardiovascular care, *Circulation* 112(suppl IV):IV-130, 2005.

Sodium Bicarbonate—cont'd

Special Considerations	• Do not mix with parenteral drugs because of the possibility of drug inactivation or precipitation • Hyperkalemia produces ECG changes including tall, peaked (tented) T waves; widened QRS complexes, prolonged PR intervals, flattened ST segments, and flattened or absent P waves. Hyperkalemia may lead to ventricular dysrhythmias and asystole if not reversed. • Sodium bicarbonate is used in hyperkalemia to decrease serum potassium (K+) levels by temporarily shifting K+ into the intracellular fluid • Sodium bicarbonate may be administered in tricyclic antidepressant overdose with QRS prolongation or hypotension.

ACUTE CORONARY SYNDROMES

Acute coronary syndromes (ACS) are conditions caused by a similar sequence of pathologic events—a temporary or permanent blockage of a coronary artery. This sequence of events results in conditions ranging from myocardial ischemia or injury to death (necrosis) of heart muscle. The usual cause of ACS is the rupture of an atherosclerotic plaque. ACS include unstable angina, non–ST-segment elevation myocardial infarction (NSTEMI), and ST-segment elevation MI (STEMI). Sudden cardiac death can occur with any of these conditions:

- Blockage of a coronary artery by a clot may be complete or incomplete.
  - Complete blockage of a coronary artery may result in STEMI or sudden death.
  - Partial (incomplete) blockage of a coronary artery by a clot may result in no clinical signs and symptoms (silent MI), unstable angina, NSTEMI, or sudden death.

- The patient's signs, symptoms, and outcome depend on factors including:
  - Amount of heart muscle supplied by the affected artery
  - Severity and duration of myocardial ischemia
  - Electrical instability of the ischemic myocardium

ACS

- Degree and duration of coronary vessel blockage
- Presence (and extent) or absence of collateral coronary circulation

Acute Coronary Syndromes – Targeted History

Historical Information to Obtain	Notes
Patient age, gender	Important risk factors
SAMPLE	
<u>S</u>igns/Symptoms	"What prompted you to seek medical assistance today?"
<u>A</u>llergies	Medications, food, environmental causes (pollen), and products (latex)
<u>M</u>edications	Prescription and over-the-counter medications (including herbal supplements), recreational substance use History of phosphodiesterase inhibitor use in the past 24-48 hours?
<u>P</u>ast medical history	History of coronary artery disease, stable or unstable angina, MI, coronary bypass surgery, or PCI? History of high blood pressure or diabetes? Risk factors present? How many? History of bleeding problems, ulcer disease, transient ischemic attack (TIA) or stroke?
<u>L</u>ast oral intake	Time of most recent meal and fluid intake
<u>E</u>vents prior	"What were you doing when it began?"
OPQRST (pain presentation)	
<u>O</u>nset	"When did your symptoms begin?" "Did your symptoms begin suddenly or gradually?"
<u>P</u>rovocation/ <u>P</u>alliative	"Did anything bring on your discomfort?" "Does anything make it better or worse?" (Associated with breathing movement)

Acute Coronary Syndromes – Targeted History—cont'd

Quality	"How would you describe your discomfort?"
Region/Radiation/Referral	"Where is your discomfort?" (Ask the patient to point to it); "Does it go anywhere else?"
Severity	"On a scale of 0 to 10, with 0 being the least and 10 being the worst, what number would you assign your pain or discomfort?"
Timing	"Does your discomfort come and go, or is it constant?"
Presence of associated symptoms?	Nausea, vomiting, sweating, weakness, fatigue
Special Considerations	Consider possibility of potentially lethal conditions that mimic acute MI such as aortic dissection, acute pericarditis, acute myocarditis, and pulmonary embolism.

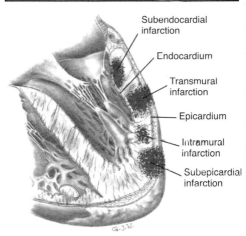

Possible locations of infarctions in the ventricular wall.[50]

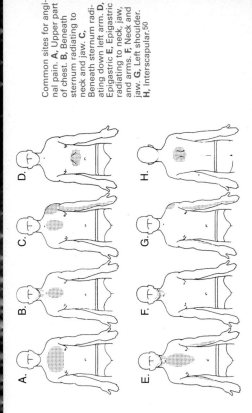

Common sites for anginal pain. **A,** Upper part of chest. **B,** Beneath sternum radiating to neck and jaw. **C,** Beneath sternum sternum radiating down left arm. **D,** Epigastric **E,** Epigastric radiating to neck, jaw, and arms. **F,** Neck and jaw. **G,** Left shoulder. **H,** Interscapular.50

The sudden blockage of a coronary artery may result in ischemia, injury, and death of the area of the myocardium supplied by the affected artery. The area supplied by the blocked artery goes through a characteristic sequence of events that have been identified as "zones" of ischemia, injury, and infarction. Each zone is associated with characteristic ECG changes. The ECG changes described below are not seen in every lead. They appear only in leads looking at the area fed by the blocked vessel. Because most infarctions occur in the left ventricle and a standard 12-lead ECG views the surfaces of the left ventricle from 12 different angles, obtain a 12-lead ECG as quickly as possible (goal is within 10 minutes of patient contact) in a patient experiencing a possible ACS.

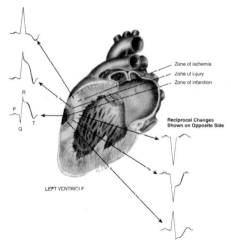

Zones of ischemia, injury, and infarction showing ECG waveforms and reciprocal waveforms corresponding to each zone.[50]

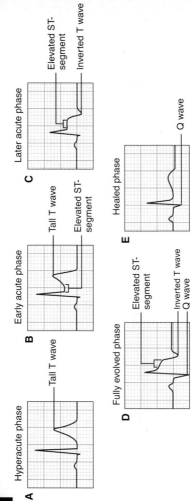

The evolving pattern of ST-elevation myocardial infarction on the ECG.[51]

A Hyperacute phase — Tall T wave

B Early acute phase — Tall T wave, Elevated ST-segment

C Later acute phase — Elevated ST-segment, Inverted T wave

D Fully evolved phase — Elevated ST-segment, Inverted T wave, Q wave

E Healed phase — Q wave

■ INDICATIVE ECG CHANGES ■

- The left ventricle has been divided into regions where a myocardial infarction may occur—septal, anterior, lateral, inferior, and posterior. In the standard 12-lead ECG, leads II, III, and aVF "look" at tissue supplied by the right coronary artery. A total of 8 leads "look" at tissue supplied by the left coronary artery: leads I, aVL, V_1, V_2, V_3, V_4, V_5, and V_6. When evaluating the extent of infarction produced by a left coronary artery occlusion, decide how many of these leads are showing indicative changes. The more of these 8 leads that show indicative changes, the larger the infarction is presumed to be.[3]

- Indicative ECG changes are significant when they are seen in at least two *contiguous* leads. Two leads are contiguous if they look at the same or adjacent area of the heart or they are numerically consecutive chest leads.

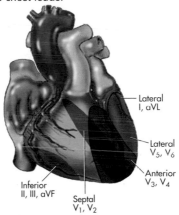

Lateral
I, aVL

Lateral
V_5, V_6

Anterior
V_3, V_4

Inferior
II, III, aVF

Septal
V_1, V_2

The surfaces of the heart. The posterior surface is not shown.[52]

Localizing ECG changes

I Lateral	aVR _____	V₁ Septum	V₄ Anterior	V₄R Right Ventricle
II Inferior	aVL Lateral	V₂ Septum	V₅ Lateral	V₅R Right Ventricle
III Inferior	aVF Inferior	V₃ Anterior	V₆ Lateral	V₆R Right Ventricle

▣ EVALUATING THE 12-LEAD ECG ▣

Obtaining and reviewing a 12-lead ECG is an important component of the initial assessment of the patient with ischemic chest discomfort. Obtain the first 12-lead ECG within 10 minutes of patient contact or the patient's arrival in the emergency department. Repeat with each set of vital signs, when the patient's symptoms change, and as often as necessary.

Once the 12-lead has been obtained in a patient experiencing an ACS, it should be reviewed carefully. Look at each lead for the presence of ST-segment displacement (elevation or depression). If ST-segment elevation is present, note its elevation in millimeters. Examine the T waves for any changes in orientation, shape, and size. Examine each lead for the presence of a Q wave. If a Q wave is present, measure its duration. Assess the areas of ischemia or injury by assessing lead groupings. Remember: ECG evidence must be found in at least two contiguous leads.

Based on the 12-lead ECG findings, categorize the patient into one of three groups:

- *ST-segment elevation.* ST-segment elevation in two or more contiguous leads or new-onset left bundle branch block suggests myocardial injury. This patient is classified as STEMI. Patients with obvious ST elevation in leads II, III, and/or aVF should also be evaluated for possible right ventricular MI. Patients with ST elevation in two or more contiguous leads should be evaluated for immediate reperfusion therapy.

- *ST-segment depression.* ST depression or transient ST/T-wave changes that occur with pain or discomfort suggest myocardial ischemia. This patient is classified as high-risk UA/NSTEMI. Patients with obvious ST depression in leads V_1 and V_2 should be evaluated for possible posterior MI. The patient with high-risk UA/NSTEMI should be admitted to a monitored bed for further evaluation.

- *Normal/nondiagnostic ECG.* A normal ECG or nonspecific ST- and T-wave changes are nondiagnostic and should prompt consideration for further evaluation. Consider admission of the patient with signs and symptoms suggesting an ACS and a non-diagnostic ECG to the emergency department chest pain unit or to an appropriate bed. Obtain cardiac biomarkers on initial presentation and again between 6 and 12 hours after symptom onset. Obtaining serial ECGs at 5- to 10-minute intervals or continuous ST-segment monitoring should be performed.

Bundle branch block, left ventricular hypertrophy, an idioventricular rhythm, or a paced rhythm may make the ECG signs of ischemia or injury difficult or impossible to interpret. An absence of signs of ischemia, injury, or infarction on an ECG or in early laboratory data does not exclude the possibility of an ACS.

Localization of a Myocardial Infarction

Location of MI	Indicative Changes (Leads facing affected area)	Affected Coronary Artery
Anterior	V_3, V_4	Left coronary artery • LAD – diagonal branch
Anteroseptal	V_1, V_2, V_3, V_4	Left coronary artery • LAD – diagonal branch • LAD – septal branch
Anterolateral	I, aVL, V_3, V_4, V_5, V_6	Left coronary artery • LAD – diagonal branch and/or • Circumflex branch
Inferior	II, III, aVF	Right coronary artery (most common) – posterior descending branch or left coronary artery (circumflex branch)
Lateral	I, aVL, V_5, V_6	Left coronary artery • LAD – diagonal branch and/or • Circumflex branch Right coronary artery
Septum	V_1, V_2	Left coronary artery • LAD – septal branch
Posterior	V_7, V_8, V_9	Right coronary or left circumflex artery
Right Ventricle	V_1R-V_6R	Right coronary artery • Proximal branches

ROUTINE MEASURES (MONA)

OXYGEN

Supplemental oxygen administration is indicated if the patient is hypoxic, cyanotic, having difficulty breathing, has obvious signs of heart failure or shock, or if his oxygen saturation declines to less than 94%. Titrate oxygen therapy to maintain the patient's SpO_2 at 94% or greater.

ASPIRIN

- Give 162- to 325-mg of nonenteric aspirin as soon as possible after symptom onset, if there are no contraindications.
- Chewable aspirin allows for quicker absorption.
- Flavored chewable aspirin may be better accepted by the patient over standard aspirin tablets.

NITROGLYCERIN (NTG)

- NTG relaxes vascular smooth muscle, including dilation of the coronary arteries (particularly in the area of plaque disruption). It also decreases myocardial oxygen consumption.
- Before giving NTG, make sure an IV is in place, the patient's systolic blood pressure is greater than 90 mm Hg, heart rate is between 50 and 100 beats/minute, there are no signs of right ventricular infarction, and the patient has not used a phosphodiesterase inhibitor in the previous 24 to 48 hours.
- NTG SL tablets or spray may be given at 5 minute intervals to a maximum of 3 doses if discomfort persists and vital signs remain stable.
- Consider the presence of right ventricular infarction if the patient with an inferior wall infarction becomes hypotensive after administration of nitrates.

MORPHINE

- Morphine is the preferred analgesic for patients with STEMI who experience persistent chest discomfort unresponsive to nitrates.

- Morphine is reasonable for non-ST elevation patients whose symptoms are not relieved despite NTG (e.g., after serial sublingual NTG tablets) or whose symptoms recur despite adequate anti-ischemic therapy.

ADULT STROKE

There are two major types of stroke—ischemic and hemorrhagic. An ischemic stroke occurs when a blood vessel supplying the brain is blocked. It can be life-threatening but rarely leads to death within the first hour. A hemorrhagic stroke occurs when a cerebral artery bursts. It can be fatal at onset.

The time from onset of stroke symptoms until treatment is a key factor for success of any therapy. The earlier the treatment for stroke, the more favorable the results are likely to be. Blood flow needs to be restored to the affected area as quickly as possible. Intravenous administration of a recombinant form of tPA (tissue plasminogen activator) (rtPA) has proved to be an effective cerebral reperfusion therapy. Currently, the window of opportunity to use IV rtPA to treat ischemic stroke patients is within 3 hours of symptom onset.

Direct administration of intra-arterial (IA) fibrinolytic agents into the clot, while passing the catheter through the clot and mechanically disrupting it has been pursued as an alternative strategy to treat selected patients who have a large stroke of less than 6 hours duration secondary to occlusion of the middle cerebral artery and who are not otherwise candidates for IV rtPA (such as recent surgery). Because intra-arterial therapy requires access to emergent cerebral angiography, experienced stroke physicians, and neurointerventionalists, it should be performed only at an experienced center.

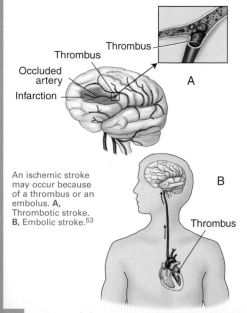

An ischemic stroke may occur because of a thrombus or an embolus. **A,** Thrombotic stroke. **B,** Embolic stroke.[53]

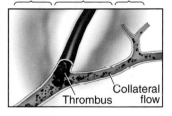

Penumbra   Infarction   Penumbra

Collateral flow

Thrombus

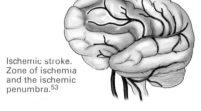

Ischemic stroke. Zone of ischemia and the ischemic penumbra.[53]

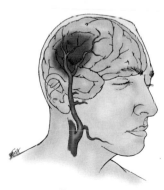

Hemorrhagic stroke.[54]

Signs and Symptoms of Stroke

Affected Artery	Structures Supplied by Affected Vessel	Signs and Symptoms of Blockage
Anterior cerebral	Supplies medial surfaces and upper portions of frontal and parietal lobes	Emotional lability Confusion Weakness, numbness on affected side Paralysis of contralateral foot and leg Impaired mobility, with sensation greater in lower extremities than in upper Urinary incontinence Loss of coordination Personality changes Impaired sensory function
Middle cerebral (Most commonly blocked vessel in stroke) (Largest branch of the internal carotid artery)	Supplies a portion of the frontal lobe, lateral surface of the temporal and parietal lobes, including the primary motor and sensory areas of the face, throat, hand, and arm and in the dominant hemisphere, the areas for speech	Changes in communication, cognition, mobility, and sensation including: Aphasia Dysphasia Reading difficulty (dyslexia) Inability to write (dysgraphia) Visual field deficits

Posterior cerebral	Supplies medial and inferior temporal lobes, medial occipital lobe, thalamus, posterior hypothalamus, visual receptive area	Contralateral sensory deficit Contralateral hemiparesis (more severe in the face and hand than in the leg) Altered level of responsiveness Hemiplegia Receptive aphasia Sensory impairment Dyslexia Coma Visual field deficits Cortical blindness from ischemia
Internal carotid	Supplies cerebral hemispheres and diencephalon	Headaches Altered level of responsiveness Bruits over the carotid artery Profound aphasia Ptosis Weakness, paralysis, numbness, sensory changes, and visual deficits (blurring) on the affected side Unilateral blindness

Continued.

Signs and Symptoms of Stroke—cont'd

Affected Artery	Structures Supplied by Affected Vessel	Signs and Symptoms of Blockage
Vertebral or basilar	Supplies brainstem and cerebellum	*Incomplete blockage* Transient ischemic attacks Unilateral and bilateral weakness of extremities Visual deficits on affected side (diplopia, color blindness, lack of depth perception) Nausea, vertigo, tinnitus Headache Dysarthria Numbness Dysphagia "Locked-in" syndrome—no movement except eyelids; sensation and consciousness preserved *Complete blockage* Coma Extension (decerebrate) posturing Respiratory and circulatory abnormalities

CINCINNATI PREHOSPITAL STROKE SCALE

Facial droop/weakness: Ask patient to "Show me your teeth" or "Smile for me"
- Normal: Both sides of face move equally well
- Abnormal: One side of face does not move at all

Motor weakness (arm drift): With eyes closed, ask patient to extend arms out in front of him or her 90° (if sitting) or 45° (if supine). Drift is scored if the arm falls before 10 seconds have elapsed.
- Normal: Both arms move the same OR both arms do not move at all
- Abnormal: One arm either does not move OR one arm drifts down compared to the other

Aphasia (speech): Ask the patient to say "A rolling stone gathers no moss, You can't teach an old dog new tricks, The sky is blue in Cincinnati," or a similar phrase
- Normal: Phrase is repeated clearly and correctly
- Abnormal: Patient uses inappropriate words, words are slurred (dysarthria), or the patient is unable to talk

If any one of these signs is abnormal, stroke probability is 72%

INITIAL EMERGENCY CARE

Within 10 minutes of the patient's arrival:
- Reassess the patient's ABCs and take the patient's vital signs.
- Check the patient's oxygen saturation level and give oxygen if the patient is hypoxemic (SpO_2 below 94%) or if the patient's oxygen saturation is unknown.

- Make sure that an IV has been established. Avoid dextrose-containing solutions because they can increase swelling of the brain.
- Check the patient's blood sugar level and treat if indicated. Give dextrose if the patient is hypoglycemic. Administration of insulin is recommended if the patient's serum glucose is more than 185 mg/dL in a patient with acute stroke.
- Obtain a 12-lead ECG and assess for dysrhythmias.
- Perform a general neurologic screening assessment and alert the stroke team: neurologist, radiologist, and computed tomography (CT) technician.

NINDS-Recommended Stroke Evaluation Targets for Potential Fibrinolytic Candidates	
Activity	**Target**
Door to physician evaluation	10 minutes
Door to access to neurological expertise (in person or by phone)	15 minutes
Door to CT completion	25 minutes
Door to CT read	45 minutes
Door to drug/intervention	60 minutes
Door to neurosurgical availability (on-site or by transport)	2 hours
Door to admission to monitored bed	3 hours

Within 25 minutes of the patient's arrival:
- Review the patient's history
- Verify the time of symptom onset (less than 3 hours required for IV fibrinolytics). When was the last time the patient was known to be without symptoms? What was the patient doing when the symptoms began? Did the patient complain of a

headache? Did a seizure occur? Has there been a change in the level of responsiveness? Is there a history of any recent trauma?

- Review the patient's medical history. Determine the presence of stroke risk factors. Find out the medications the patient is currently taking and the patient's allergies to medications.
- Perform a physical exam.
- Perform a neurologic exam. Scales are used in order to give quantifiable information to other members of the stroke team.
  ‣ Use the Glasgow Coma Scale (GCS) to determine level of responsiveness. The GCS measures impairment but is of limited use in an intubated patient, a patient with orbital trauma, or a patient with previous neurological impairment.
  ‣ Use the National Institutes of Health Stroke Scale (NIHSS) to determine the severity of the stroke. The NIHSS is used to assess neurologic outcome and degree of recovery. Use of this scale allows a standardized way to assess outcome and compare outcomes with other centers. The NIHSS is usually performed by a neurologist and takes roughly 7 minutes to perform. Treatment should not be delayed by using this scale.
- Diagnostic studies that should be obtained in all patients with suspected acute ischemic stroke include the following:
  ‣ Urgent, noncontrast CT scan or brain MRI.
  ‣ ECG, serum glucose, serum electrolytes, cardiac biomarkers
  ‣ Complete blood count, including platelet count
  ‣ Renal function, prothrombin and partial thromboplastin times

- Additional diagnostic studies should be obtained in selected cases such as pregnancy testing, blood alcohol level, urine or blood toxicology screen (for patients with possible substance abuse), liver function tests and ammonia level (for patients with an unexplained altered level of consciousness), lumbar puncture (for suspected meningitis or if subarachnoid hemorrhage is suspected and CT is negative for blood), electroencephalogram (for suspected seizures), and arterial blood gas tests (for suspected hypoxia).
- A 12-lead ECG should be obtained to evaluate for pre-existing cardiac disease and concurrent myocardial injury.
- A chest radiograph should be obtained in stroke patients with dysphagia or if lung disease is suspected, and for patients with respiratory distress or hypoxia.

ELECTROLYTE ABNORMALITIES

Electrolyte disturbances are a common cause of dysrhythmias. If not corrected, electrolyte abnormalities can lead to cardiac arrest and complicate resuscitation and postresuscitation care.

POTASSIUM

Hyperkalemia
ECG changes correlate with the degree of hyperkalemia

Serum potassium level	ECG change
5.6 to 6.0 mEq/L	Tall, peaked (tented) T waves
6.0 to 6.5 mEq/L	Prolonged PR and QT intervals
6.5 to 7.0 mEq/L	P wave amplitude decreases, flattened ST-segments

7.0 to 8.0 mEq/L	P waves eventually disappear, QRS widens
8.0 to 12.0 mEq/L	Wide QRS complexes
>15.0 mEq/L	Ventricular fibrillation, asystole

Initial Emergency Care

- ABCs, O_2, IV, monitor
- Stop potassium intake (oral and IV)
- Stop all medications that might be associated with hyperkalemia (ACE inhibitors, potassium-sparing diuretics)
- Mild hyperkalemia (5 to 6 mEq/L): Remove potassium from the body with furosemide, Kayexalate
- Moderate hyperkalemia (6 to 7 mEq/L): Shift potassium into the cells with glucose plus insulin, sodium bicarbonate, or nebulized albuterol
- Severe hyperkalemia (>7 mEq/L)
  - Stabilize myocardial cell membrane with calcium chloride or calcium gluconate IV
  - Shift potassium into the cells with sodium bicarbonate, glucose plus insulin, or nebulized albuterol
  - Remove potassium from the body with furosemide, Kayexalate, or dialysis

Hypokalemia

ECG changes correlate with the degree of hypokalemia:

- T wave amplitude decreases
- T waves flatten, U waves appear
- ST-segment becomes depressed
- U waves increase in size; PR, QRS, and QT intervals lengthen

Initial Emergency Care

- ABCs, O_2, IV, monitor
- Oral potassium preferred for mild hypokalemia, IV if unable to tolerate oral therapy
- Moderate hypokalemia (2.5 to 3 mEq/L): Oral potassium preferred, IV if unable to tolerate oral therapy
- Severe hypokalemia (less than 2.5 mEq/L): IV potassium replacement

SODIUM

Hypernatremia

Hypernatremia most often occurs in very young, elderly, debilitated, or altered patients

Initial Emergency Care

- ABCs, O_2, IV, monitor
- Treat the underlying cause
- Replace fluid orally or via nasogastric tube if patient is stable and asymptomatic
- IV normal saline or a 5% dextrose in half-normal saline solution is used to restore extracellular fluid volume in hypovolemic patients

Hyponatremia

Initial Emergency Care

- ABCs, O_2, IV, monitor
- Treatment depends on the patient's volume status.
- Hypovolemic patients need oral or IV sodium. Isotonic saline is usually used initially and then changed to a hypotonic fluid, such as 0.45% saline, once hypovolemia is corrected.
- Patients with normal volume or hypervolemia are usually treated by restricting

water. With significant fluid overload, a loop diuretic may be necessary.

MAGNESIUM

Hypermagnesemia

Initial Emergency Care

- ABCs, O_2, IV, monitor
- Stop magnesium intake (oral and IV)
- Calcium chloride may be given IV if severe hypermagnesemia is present to reverse respiratory depression, hypotension, and cardiac dysrhythmias

Hypomagnesemia

Initial Emergency Care

- ABCs, O_2, IV, monitor
- For severe or symptomatic hypomagnesemia, give magnesium sulfate IV

CALCIUM

Normal values: 4.5 to 5.5 mEq/L or 9 to 11 mg/dL

Hypercalcemia

Initial Emergency Care

- ABCs, O_2, IV, monitor
- Give 0.9% saline IV to restore intravascular volume and induce diuresis
- Watch potassium and magnesium levels closely
- Patients with heart failure or renal insufficiency may need hemodialysis to rapidly decrease serum calcium

Hypocalcemia

Initial Emergency Care

- ABCs, O_2, IV, monitor
- Calcium chloride or calcium gluconate IV

- Watch magnesium, potassium, and pH closely

TOXICOLOGY

The poisoned patient may require treatment that differs from standard ACLS guidelines. It is important to recognize the signs and symptoms of poisoning and consult a clinical toxicologist/poison control center for assistance in determining an appropriate patient treatment plan. Poison Control Centers provide free, 24-hour emergency telephone access to poison experts for the public and medical professionals. 1-800-222-1222 is the telephone number for every poison center in the United States.

ASSESSMENT OF THE PATIENT WITH A POSSIBLE TOXIC EXPOSURE

History

The history provides critical information in the assessment of the patient with a suspected toxic exposure. In addition to a SAMPLE history, critical questions to ask in a toxic exposure situation include what, when, where, why, and how.

- What is the poison?
  - ‣ Determine the exact name of the product, if possible
  - ‣ Obtain histories from different family members to help confirm the type and dose of exposure.
  - ‣ Any pill bottles, commercial products, or plants seen support the history?
- How was it taken (ingested, inhaled, absorbed, or injected)?
- When was it taken?
  - ‣ Knowing the time of ingestion is critical when considering gastric emptying and antidote administration.
- Where was the patient found? Were there

any witnesses or any other people around?

- How much was taken?
  ‣ How many pills, how much liquid was taken?
  ‣ How many (amount) were available before ingestion?
  ‣ How many (much) are now in the container?
- Where is the substance stored?
- What is the patient's age? Weight?
- Has the patient vomited? How many times?
- What home remedies have been tried? (Ask about herbal or folk remedies.)
- Has a Poison Control Center been contacted? If so, what instructions were received? What treatment has already been given?
- Has the patient been depressed or experienced recent emotional stress?

Focused Physical Examination

When performing a physical examination on a patient with a known or suspected toxic exposure, be alert in your search for information regarding the severity and cause of the exposure. Changes in the patient's mental status, vital signs, skin temperature and moisture, and pupil size may provide a collection of physical findings typical of a specific toxin. Characteristic findings that are useful in recognizing a specific class of poisoning are called a toxidrome. Your physical examination findings may provide the only clues to the presence of a toxin if the patient is unresponsive. Familiarity with common toxidromes helps in to recognizing the diagnostic significance of the patient history and physical examination findings and implementing an appropriate treatment plan.

Clinical Presentations of Specific Toxidromes

Toxidrome	Signs/Symptoms	Typical Agents	Primary Antidote
Anticholinergic	Agitation or reduced responsiveness, tachypnea, tachycardia, slightly elevated temperature, blurred vision, dilated pupils, urinary retention, decreased bowel sounds; dry, flushed skin	Atropine, diphenhydramine, scopolamine	Physostigmine
Cholinergic	Altered mental status, tachypnea, bronchospasm, bradycardia or tachycardia, salivation, constricted pupils, polyuria, defecation, emesis, fever, lacrimation, seizures, diaphoresis	Organophosphate insecticides (malathion), carbamate insecticides (carbaryl), some mushrooms, nerve agents	Atropine
Opioid	Altered mental status, bradypnea or apnea, bradycardia, hypotension, pinpoint pupils, hypothermia	Codeine, fentanyl, heroin, meperidine, methadone, oxycodone, dextromethorphan, propoxyphene	Naloxone

Sedative/Hypnotic	Slurred speech, confusion, hypotension, tachycardia, pupil dilation or constriction, dry mouth, respiratory depression, decreased temperature, delirium, hallucinations, coma, paresthesias, blurred vision, ataxia, nystagmus	Ethanol, anticonvulsants, barbiturates, benzodiazepines	Benzodiazepines: flumazenil
Sympathomimetic	Agitation, tachypnea, tachycardia, hypertension, excessive speech and motor activity, tremor, dilated pupils, disorientation, insomnia, psychosis, fever, seizures, diaphoresis	Albuterol, amphetamines (e.g., "ecstasy"), caffeine, cocaine, epinephrine, ephedrine, methamphetamine, phencyclidine, pseudoephedrine	Benzodiazepines

Toxicology Memory Aids

Anticholinergic Syndrome (antihistamines, tricyclic antidepressants)	• Mad as a hatter–confused, delirium • Red as a beet–flushed skin • Dry as a bone–dry mouth • Hot as Hades–hyperthermia • Blind as a bat–dilated pupils
Cholinergic Syndrome ("SLUDGE" or "DUMBELS")	• **S**alivation, **L**acrimation, **U**rination, **D**efecation, **G**astrointestinal distress, **E**mesis • **D**iarrhea, **U**rination, **M**iosis (pinpoint pupils), **B**ronchospasm / **B**ronchorrhea / **B**radycardia, **E**mesis, **L**acrimation, **S**alivation

Odors and Toxins

Odor	Toxin
Acetone	Acetone, isopropyl alcohol, salicylates
Alcohol	Ethanol, isopropyl alcohol
Bitter almonds	Cyanide
Carrots	Water hemlock
Fishy	Zinc or aluminum phosphide
Fruity	Isopropyl alcohol, chlorinated hydrocarbons (e.g., chloroform)
Garlic	Arsenic, organophosphates, phosphorus, thallium
Glue	Toluene
Mothballs	Camphor
Pears	Chloral hydrate, paraldehyde
Rotten eggs	Sulfur dioxide, hydrogen sulfide
Shoe polish	Nitrobenzene
Vinyl	Ethchlorvynol
Wintergreen	Methyl salicylates

Toxins and Vital Sign Changes

Vital Sign	Increased	Decreased
Temperature	Amphetamines, anticholinergics, antihistamines, antipsychotic agents, cocaine, monoamine oxidase inhibitors, nicotine, phenothiazines, salicylates, sympathomimetics, theophylline, tricyclic antidepressants, serotonin reuptake inhibitors	Barbiturates, carbon monoxide, clonidine, ethanol, insulin, opiates, oral hypoglycemic agents, phenothiazines, sedative/hypnotics
Pulse	Amphetamines, anticholinergics, antihistamines, cocaine, phencyclidine, sympathomimetics, theophylline	Alcohol, beta-blockers, calcium channel blockers, carbamates, clonidine, cardiac glycosides, opiates, organophosphates
Ventilations	Amphetamines, barbiturates (early), caffeine, cocaine, ethylene glycol, methanol, salicylates	Alcohols and ethanol, barbiturates (late), clonidine, opiates, sedative/hypnotics
Blood Pressure	Amphetamines, anticholinergics, antihistamines, caffeine, clonidine, cocaine, marijuana, phencyclidine, sympathomimetics, theophylline	Antihypertensives, barbiturates, beta-blockers, calcium channel blockers, clonidine, cyanide, opiates, phenothiazines, sedative/hypnotics, tricyclic antidepressants (late)

DROWNING

INITIAL EMERGENCY CARE FOR DROWNING

- Remove the victim from the water as quickly as possible while ensuring rescuer safety.

- Oxygenation and ventilation are is the most important treatments for a drowning victim. Start rescue breathing as soon as the victim's airway can be opened and the rescuer's safety can be ensured (usually when the victim is in shallow water or out of the water). Consider mouth-to-nose ventilation if it is difficult to perform mouth-to-mouth ventilation while the victim is in the water.

- The airway does not need to be cleared of aspirated water; however, debris, gastric contents, or other foreign material may need to be removed. The routine use of abdominal thrusts or the Heimlich maneuver to remove water from the breathing passages is not recommended. Instead, suctioning should be used for this purpose when indicated.

- After removal from the water, begin rescue breathing if the victim is apneic (if not already started while the victim was in the water). If a pulse cannot be felt or you are unsure if a pulse is present, begin chest compressions. It may be difficult to feel a pulse because of peripheral vasoconstriction and decreased cardiac output. Attach an AED and defibrillate if a shockable rhythm is identified.

- The victim should be transported to the closest appropriate facility for evaluation and monitoring.

INITIAL STABILIZATION

Assess the asthma patient's mental status, ability to complete a sentence (age dependent), presence of a cough, breathlessness, and chest tightness. Assess pulse rate, ventilatory rate, breath sounds, use of accessory muscles, and presence of suprasternal retractions. Close monitoring is essential. Initial stabilization of the patient who has life-threatening asthma includes the use of oxygen, bronchodilators, and steroids. A pulmonologist or intensivist should be consulted if the patient does not respond to treatment.

- Give oxygen to all patients (including those with normal oxygenation) to maintain an oxygen saturation of 94% or higher.
- Give a short-acting beta$_2$-agonist, such as albuterol. Continuous administration may be more effective than intermittent administration.
- To reduce inflammation, asthma patients should receive systemic corticosteroids as early as possible, although the effects may not be evident for several hours. Because patients with near-fatal asthma may vomit or be unable to swallow, the IV route is preferred.

ADJUNCTIVE THERAPY[8]

- Anticholinergics
  - Ipratropium bromide
    - Anticholinergic bronchodilator
    - Slow onset of action (about 20 minutes), peak effects at 60 to 90 minutes
    - Consider as an adjunct to albuterol

- Magnesium sulfate
  - Causes bronchial smooth muscle relaxation
  - When given IV, can improve pulmonary function when combined with nebulized beta agonists and corticosteroids
  - Nebulized magnesium sulfate may also improve pulmonary function in acute asthma when given with a B_2-agonist
- Parenteral epinephrine or terbutaline
  - Can be given SubQ to patients with acute severe asthma
  - SubQ epinephrine is given in three divided doses about 20 minutes apart. Use 1:1000 concentration.
  - Terbutaline is given SubQ and can be repeated every 20 minutes for 3 doses.
- Ketamine
  - Dissociative anesthetic with bronchodilatory properties
  - Can stimulate copious bronchial secretions
- Heliox
  - Mixture of helium and oxygen (usually a 70:30 helium to oxygen ratio mix)
  - Has been shown to improve delivery and deposition of nebulized albuterol
  - If the patient needs more than 30% oxygen, heliox cannot be used
- Methylxanthines: Infrequently used due to erratic pharmacokinetics and adverse effects
- Leukotriene antagonists: Effectiveness during acute asthma exacerbations unproven
- Inhaled anesthetics
  - Sevoflurane and isoflurane may have bronchodilator effects
  - Use increases the ease of mechanical ventilation and reduces oxygen demand and carbon dioxide production

‣ Additional studies needed to evaluate effectiveness

ASSISTED VENTILATION[9]

- Use of noninvasive positive pressure ventilation (NIPPV), such as bilevel positive airway pressure (BiPAP), for patients with acute respiratory failure may delay or eliminate the need for tracheal intubation.
- Intubation and positive-pressure ventilation can trigger further bronchoconstriction and complications such as breath stacking and barotrauma. Breath stacking can lead to hyperinflation, tension pneumothorax, and hypotension.
  ‣ Manual and mechanical ventilation differs from that provided to nonasthmatic patients:
    - Use slower ventilatory rate with smaller tidal volumes (6 to 8 mL/kg)
    - Use shorter inspiratory time (adult inspiratory flow rate 80 to 100 mL/min)
    - Use longer expiratory time (inspiratory to expiratory ratio 1:4 or 1:5)
- Perform elective intubation if the asthmatic patient deteriorates despite aggressive therapy:
  ‣ Rapid sequence intubation is technique of choice
  ‣ To decrease airway resistance, use the largest tracheal tube available
  ‣ Confirm tube placement after insertion
  ‣ Sedation may be needed after intubation
- If the patient deteriorates or become difficult to ventilate after intubation, use the DOPE memory aid to troubleshoot
  ‣ **D**isplaced tube (right mainstem or esophageal intubation)—Reassess tube position
  ‣ **O**bstructed tube (secretions obstructing

air flow)—Suction

- ► **P**neumothorax (tension)—Needle thoracostomy
- ► **E**quipment problem/failure—Check equipment and oxygen source

ANAPHYLAXIS

INITIAL EMERGENCY CARE[10]

- ABCs, O_2, IV, cardiac monitor, pulse oximeter
- Give epinephrine intramuscularly (use 1:1000 solution) early to all patients who have signs of a systemic reaction, especially hypotension, airway swelling, or difficulty breathing. The use of an epinephrine autoinjector is recommended (if available) in both anaphylaxis and cardiac arrest with associated anaphylaxis.
- Advanced airway management, including a surgical airway, may be necessary if the patient develops hoarseness, lingual edema, stridor, or oropharyngeal swelling.
- Repeated boluses of isotonic crystalloid titrated to a systolic blood pressure of higher than 90 mm Hg may be necessary if hypotension is present and is unresponsive to vasoactive medications. Repeat the primary survey after each fluid bolus. Monitor closely for increased work of breathing and the development of crackles.
- The use of antihistamines, inhaled beta-agonists, and IV corticosteroids may be considered in the management of anaphylaxis and cardiac arrest with associated anaphylaxis.

HYPOTHERMIA

Hypothermia may result from a decrease in heat production, an increase in heat loss, or a combination of these factors. Hypothermia may be divided into three categories:

- Mild (more than 93.2° to 96.8° F [34° to 36° C])
- Moderate (86° to 93.2° F [30° to 34° C])
- Severe (less than 86° F [30° C])

INITIAL EMERGENCY CARE[11]

- Emergency care depends on the degree of heat loss.
- Passive external rewarming (appropriate for all types of hypothermia) includes moving the patient to a warm environment, removal of wet garments, and application of warm, dry clothing and blankets. Generally, this form of rewarming is adequate for the mildly hypothermic patient.
- The patient who is moderately hypothermic and has a perfusing rhythm will generally require active external rewarming, which includes the application of radiant heat, warm air, or heat packs.
- The severely hypothermic patient who has a perfusing rhythm may require active internal (core) rewarming techniques such as warm-water lavage of the chest cavity or extracorporeal rewarming through partial cardiopulmonary bypass but rewarming success has been reported with active external warming methods. The severely hypothermic patient in cardiac arrest can be rapidly rewarmed using active internal rewarming techniques. Slower rewarming techniques, such as administration of warmed humidified oxygen and warmed

parenteral fluids given via the intravenous or intraosseous (IO) routes, may be used in addition to active rewarming methods.

- Airway management procedures and establishing vascular access should not be delayed.

- Begin CPR if the hypothermic victim is pulseless and apneic. Begin rescue breathing if the victim is apneic but a pulse is present.

- If the hypothermic patient is in cardiac arrest and VT or VF is present, attempt defibrillation.

- It may be reasonable to consider vasopressor administration during hypothermic cardiac arrest according to standard ACLS cardiac arrest guidelines in combination with rewarming methods.

- If there is a return of spontaneous circulation (and if appropriate), rewarm the patient to approximately 32° to 34°C, which is consistent with current ACLS post-cardiac arrest guidelines.

TRAUMATIC CARDIAC ARREST

Cardiac arrests due to blunt trauma have a higher mortality rate than cardiac arrests due to penetrating trauma. Possible reversible causes of traumatic cardiac arrest include hypoxia, hypovolemia, pneumothorax or pericardial tamponade, and hypothermia.

INITIAL EMERGENCY CARE

- Use a jaw thrust without head tilt maneuver to open the airway. When possible, use a second rescuer to manually stabilize head and neck until full spinal stabilization can be accomplished.
- Clear the airway of secretions with suctioning as needed.

- Assist breathing if ventilations are absent or inadequate. Continued manual stabilization of the head and neck by a second rescuer is needed when ventilation is provided with a barrier device, a pocket face mask, or a bag-mask device. Each ventilation should be delivered with enough force to produce gentle chest rise. Consider the possibility of a flail chest, tension pneumothorax, or hemothorax if the chest does not rise during ventilation despite an open airway.
- Stop any obvious hemorrhage using direct pressure and dressings. Begin CPR and defibrillate if indicated.
- Advanced airway insertion should be considered if bag-mask ventilation is inadequate. Maintain manual in-line stabilization of the head and neck during the procedure. If appropriately trained rescuers are available, cricothyrotomy should be considered if advanced airway insertion is not possible/unsuccessful and inadequate ventilation persists.
- After ensuring that the patient's airway is open and oxygenation and ventilation are adequate, establish vascular access to replace lost vascular volume.
- Search for reversible causes of the cardiac arrest.

▌ CARDIAC ARREST AND PREGNANCY ▌

INITIAL EMERGENCY CARE

- The weight of the pregnant uterus on the inferior vena cava and aorta can hinder venous return and cardiac output (supine hypotension). To shift the weight of the uterus off these major blood vessels, place a patient who is 20 weeks pregnant or more and critically ill 27° to 30° back from the left lateral position (left-lateral tilt).

- If the patient experiences a cardiac arrest, alert the maternal cardiac arrest team as soon as possible and document the time of onset of the arrest. The patient may first be placed in a supine position and the gravid uterus manually displaced to the left using one or two hands. If this technique is unsuccessful, the left-lateral tilt may be used but may result in less forceful chest compressions than are possible with the patient in a supine position. Placement of a wedge, rolled blanket, or other object under the patient's right hip and chest may help maintain the left-lateral tilt position. An immediate emergency cesarean section should be considered if chest compressions remain inadequate after attempting these positions.

- Support oxygenation and ventilation and perform bag-mask ventilation with 100% oxygen. Monitor the patient's oxygen saturation closely. Because the gravid uterus causes elevation of the patient's diaphragm and abdominal contents, it may be necessary to ventilate using less volume.

- To compensate for the patient's elevated diaphragm, chest compressions should be performed slightly higher on the sternum than normally recommended in adult cardiac arrest. It is not necessary to modify energy settings or pad/paddle position if defibrillation is required. Before delivering a shock, remove internal or external fetal monitors (if present).

- Establish IV access above the diaphragm and give ACLS medications without modification during cardiac arrest.

- Consider possible reversible causes of the

cardiac arrest and provide appropriate post-cardiac arrest care.

ELECTRIC SHOCK OR LIGHTNING STRIKE

INITIAL EMERGENCY CARE

- Make certain that the scene is safe to enter before approaching the victim. Begin appropriate BLS care if spontaneous breathing or circulation is absent.

- Remove smoldering clothing, belts, and shoes. Assume cardiac arrest involving electricity is also associated with trauma until proven otherwise; protect the cervical spine and treat associated injuries as time permits.

- Treat dysrhythmias per the ACLS guidelines for these rhythms.

- Advanced airway placement may be difficult in patients with electrical burns of the face, mouth, or anterior neck because of soft tissue swelling.

- If there is a return of spontaneous circulation and significant tissue destruction is present, rapid IV fluid administration is warranted to counteract shock, correct ongoing fluid losses, and maintain a diuresis to avoid renal shutdown due to myoglobinuria.

- If a lightning strike involves multiple victims, the highest priority patients are those who are in respiratory or cardiac arrest ("reverse triage"). All victims of a lightning strike should be evaluated by a physician.

GOALS OF THE RESUSCITATION TEAM

Regardless of where a cardiac arrest occurs, the goals of the resuscitation team are to restore spontaneous breathing and circulation and preserve vital organ function throughout the resuscitation effort.

THE CRITICAL TASKS OF RESUSCITATION

Four Critical Tasks of Resuscitation

- Airway management
- Chest compressions
- ECG monitoring and defibrillation
- Vascular access and medication administration

ADULT CARDIAC ARREST [55]

Shout for Help/Activate Emergency Response

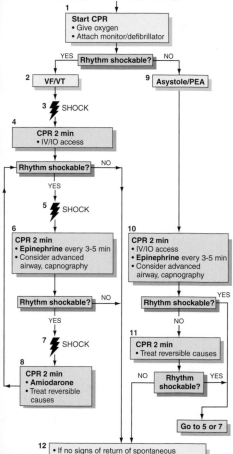

1
Start CPR
- Give oxygen
- Attach monitor/defibrillator

Rhythm shockable?
YES   NO

2 VF/VT

9 Asystole/PEA

3 ⚡ SHOCK

4
CPR 2 min
- IV/IO access

Rhythm shockable? NO

YES

5 ⚡ SHOCK

6
CPR 2 min
- **Epinephrine** every 3-5 min
- Consider advanced airway, capnography

10
CPR 2 min
- IV/IO access
- **Epinephrine** every 3-5 min
- Consider advanced airway, capnography

Rhythm shockable? NO

YES

Rhythm shockable? YES

NO

7 ⚡ SHOCK

11
CPR 2 min
- Treat reversible causes

8
CPR 2 min
- **Amiodarone**
- Treat reversible causes

Rhythm shockable?
NO   YES

Go to 5 or 7

12
- If no signs of return of spontaneous circulation (ROSC), go to **10** or **11**
- If ROSC, go to Post-Cardiac Arrest Care

CPR Quality

- Push hard (≥2 inches [5 cm]) and fast (≥100/min) and allow complete chest recoil
- Minimize interruptions in compressions
- Avoid excessive ventilation
- Rotate compressor every 2 minutes
- If no advanced airway, 30:2 compression-ventilation ratio
- Quantitative waveform capnography
  - If $PETCO_2$ <10 mm Hg, attempt to improve CPR quality
- Intra-arterial pressure
  - If relaxation phase (diastolic) pressure <20 mm Hg, attempt to improve CPR quality

Return of Spontaneous Circulation (ROSC)

- Pulse and blood pressure
- Abrupt sustained increase in $PETCO_2$ (typically ≥40 mm Hg)
- Spontaneous arterial pressure waves with intra-arterial monitoring

Shock Energy

- **Biphasic:** Manufacturer recommendation (120-200 J); if unknown use maximum available. Second and subsequent doses should be equivalent, and higher doses may be considered.
- **Monophasic:** 360 J

Drug Therapy

- **Epinephrine IV/IO Dose:**
  1 mg every 3-5 minutes
- **Vasopressin IV/IO Dose:**
  40 units can replace first or second dose of epinephrine
- **Amiodarone IV/IO Dose:**
  First Dose: 300 mg bolus.
  Second Dose: 150 mg.

Advanced Airway

- Supraglottic advanced airway or endotracheal intubation
- Waveform capnography to confirm and monitor ET tube placement
- 8-10 breaths per minute with continuous chest compressions

Reversible Causes

- **H**ypovolemia
- **H**ypoxia
- **H**ydrogen ion (acidosis)
- **H**ypo/hyperkalemia
- **H**ypothermia
- **T**ension pneumothorax
- **T**amponade, cardiac
- **T**oxins
- **T**hrombosis, pulmonary
- **T**hrombosis, coronary

ADULT IMMEDIATE POST-CARDIAC ARREST CARE [56]

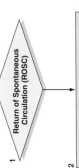

1

Return of Spontaneous Circulation (ROSC)

2

Optimize ventilation and oxygenation
- Maintain oxygen saturation ≥94%
- Consider advanced airway and waveform capnography
- Do not hyperventilate

3

Treat hypotension (SBP <90 mm Hg)
- IV/IO bolus
- Vasopressor infusion
- Consider treatable causes
- 12-Lead ECG

DOSES / DETAILS

Ventilation/Oxygenation
Avoid excessive ventilation. Start at 10-12 breaths/min and titrate to target $PETCO_2$ or 35-40 mm Hg.
When feasible, titrate FIO_2 to minimum necessary to achieve SpO_2 ≥94%.

IV Bolus
1-2 normal saline or lactated Ringer's.
If inducing hypothermia, may use 4°C fluid.

Epinephrine IV Infusion:
0.1-0.5 mcg/kg per minute (in 70-kg adult: 7-35 mcg per minute)

Dopamine IV Infusion:
5-10 mcg/kg per minute

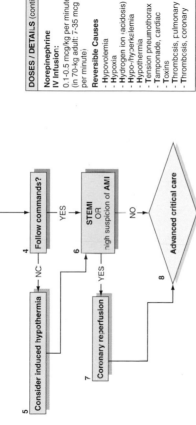

DOSES / DETAILS (continued)

Norepinephrine
IV Infusion:
0.1-0.5 mcg/kg per minute
(in 70-kg adult: 7-35 mcg
per minute)

Reversible Causes
- Hypovolemia
- Hypoxia
- Hydrogen ion (acidosis)
- Hypo-/hyperkalemia
- Hypothermia
- Tension pneumothorax
- Tamponade, cardiac
- Toxins
- Thrombosis, pulmonary
- Thrombosis, coronary

4 Follow commands?

NC

YES

5 Consider induced hypothermia

6 STEMI
OR
high suspicion of AMI

7 Coronary reperfusion

YES

NO

8 Advanced critical care

ADULT BRADYCARDIA[57]
(With Pulse)

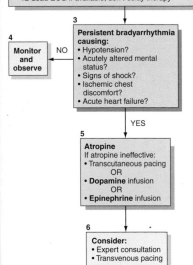

1

Assess appropriateness for clinical condition.
Heart rate typically <50/min if bradyarrhythmia.

2

Identify and treat underlying cause
- Maintain patent airway; assist breathing as necessary
- Oxygen (if hypoxemic)
- Cardiac monitor to identify rhythm; monitor blood pressure and oximetry
- IV access
- 12-Lead ECG if available; don't delay therapy

3

Persistent bradyarrhythmia causing:
- Hypotension?
- Acutely altered mental status?
- Signs of shock?
- Ischemic chest discomfort?
- Acute heart failure?

4

Monitor and observe ← NO

YES

5

Atropine
If atropine ineffective:
- Transcutaneous pacing
  OR
- **Dopamine** infusion
  OR
- **Epinephrine** infusion

6

Consider:
- Expert consultation
- Transvenous pacing

DOSES / DETAILS

Atropine IV Dose:
First dose: 0.5 mg bolus
Repeat every 3-5 minutes
Maximum: 3 mg

Dopamine IV Infusion:
2-10 mcg/kg per minute

Epinephrine IV Infusion:
2-10 mcg per minute

ADULT TACHYCARDIA [58]
(With Pulse)

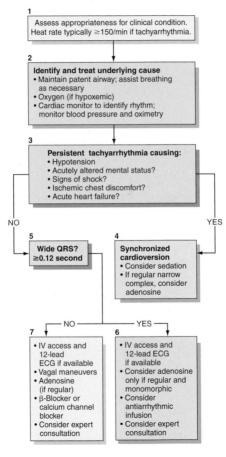

1
Assess appropriateness for clinical condition.
Heat rate typically ≥150/min if tachyarrhythmia.

2
Identify and treat underlying cause
- Maintain patent airway; assist breathing as necessary
- Oxygen (if hypoxemic)
- Cardiac monitor to identify rhythm; monitor blood pressure and oximetry

3
Persistent tachyarrhythmia causing:
- Hypotension
- Acutely altered mental status?
- Signs of shock?
- Ischemic chest discomfort?
- Acute heart failure?

NO

YES

5
Wide QRS?
≥0.12 second

4
Synchronized cardioversion
- Consider sedation
- If regular narrow complex, consider adenosine

NO

YES

7
- IV access and 12-lead ECG if available
- Vagal maneuvers
- Adenosine (if regular)
- β-Blocker or calcium channel blocker
- Consider expert consultation

6
- IV access and 12-lead ECG if available
- Consider adenosine only if regular and monomorphic
- Consider antiarrhythmic infusion
- Consider expert consultation

DOSES / DETAILS

Synchronized Cardioversion

Initial recommended doses:
- Narrow regular: 50-100 J
- Narrow irregular: 120-200 J biphasic or 200 J monophasic
- Wide regular: 100 J
- Wide irregular: defibrillation dose (Not synchronized)

Adenosine IV Dose:

First dose: 6 mg rapid IV push; follow with NS flush.
Second dose: 12 mg if required.

Antiarrhythmic Infusions for Stable Wide-QRS Tachycardia

Procainamide IV Dose:

20-50 mg/min until arrhythmia suppressed, hypotension ensues, QRS duration increases >50%, or maximum dose 17 mg/kg given.
Maintenance infusion: 1-4 mg/min.
Avoid if prolonged QT of CHF.

Amiodarone IV Dose:

First dose: 150 mg over 10 minutes.
Repeat as needed if VT recurs.
Follow by maintenance infusion of 1 mg/min for first 6 hours.

Sotalol IV Dose:

100 mg (1.5 mg/kg) over 5 minutes.
Avoid if prolonged QT.

ACUTE CORONARY SYNDROMES[59]

1

Symptoms suggestive of ischemia or infarction

2

EMS assessment and care and hospital preparation:
- Monitor, support ABCs. Be prepared to provide CPR and defibrillation
- Administer aspirin and consider oxygen, nitroglycerin, and morphine if needed
- Obtain 12-lead ECG; if ST elevation:
  – Notify receiving hospital with transmission or interpretation; note time of onset and first medical contact
- Notified hospital should mobilize hospital resources to respond to STEMI
- If considering prehospital fibrinolysis, use fibrinolytic checklist

3

Concurrent ED assessment (<10 minutes)
- Check vital signs; evaluate oxygen saturation
- Establish IV access
- Perform brief, targeted history, physical exam
- Review/complete fibrinolytic checklist; check contraindications
- Obtain initial cardiac marker levels, initial electrolyte and coagulation studies
- Obtain portable chest x-ray (<30 minutes)

Immediate ED general treatment
- If O₂ sat <94%, start **oxygen** at 4 L/min, titrate
- **Aspirin** 160 to 325 mg (if not given by EMS)
- **Nitroglycerin** sublingual or spray
- **Morphine** IV if discomfort not relieved by nitroglycerin

4
ECG interpretation

5
ST elevation or new or presumably new LBBB; strongly suspicious for injury
ST-elevation MI (STEMI)

9
ST depression or dynamic T-wave inversion; strongly suspicious for ischemia
High risk unstable angina/
non-ST-elevation MI (UA/NSTEM)

13
Normal or nondiagnostic changes in ST segment or T wave
Low-/intermediate-risk ACS

Chart Continued on Next Page

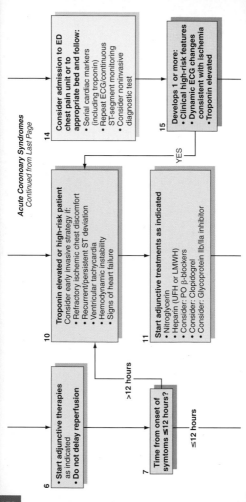

Acute Coronary Syndromes
Continued from Last Page

6
• Start adjunctive therapies as indicated
• **Do not delay reperfusion**

7
Time from onset of symtoms ≤12 hours?

>12 hours

≤12 hours

10
Troponin elevated or high-risk patient
Consider early invasive strategy if:
• Refractory ischemic chest discomfort
• Recurrent/persistent ST deviation
• Ventricular tachycardia
• Hemodynamic instability
• Signs of heart failure

11
Start adjunctive treatments as indicated
• Nitroglycerin
• Heparin (UFH or LMWH)
• Consider: PO β-blockers
• Consider: Clopidogrel
• Consider: Glycoprotein IIb/IIa inhibitor

14
Consider admission to ED chest pain unit or to appropriate bed and follow:
• Serial cardiac markers (including troponin)
• Repeat ECG/continuous ST-segment monitoring
• Consider noninvasive diagnostic test

15
Develops 1 or more:
• **Clinical high-risk features**
• **Dynamic ECG changes consistent with ischemia**
• **Troponin elevated**

YES

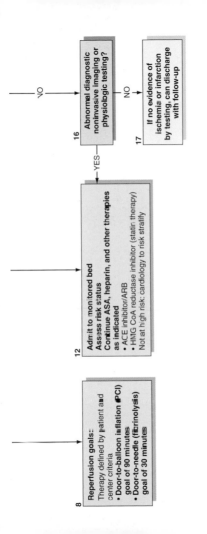

8

Reperfusion goals:
Therapy defined by patient and center criteria
• Door-to-balloon inflation (PCI) goal of 90 minutes
• Door-to-needle (fibrinolysis) goal of 30 minutes

12

Admit to monitored bed
Assess risk status
Continue ASA, heparin, and other therapies as indicated
• ACE inhibitor/ARB
• HMG CoA reductase inhibitor (statin therapy)
Not at high risk: cardiology to risk stratify

NO

16

Abnormal diagnostic noninvasive imaging or physiologic testing?

YES

NO

17

If no evidence of ischemia or infarction by testing, can discharge with follow-up

ADULT SUSPECTED STROKE [60]

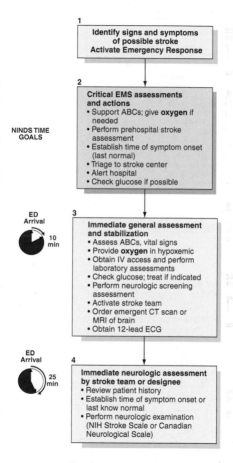

1

Identify signs and symptoms of possible stroke Activate Emergency Response

NINDS TIME GOALS

2

Critical EMS assessments and actions
- Support ABCs; give **oxygen** if needed
- Perform prehospital stroke assessment
- Establish time of symptom onset (last normal)
- Triage to stroke center
- Alert hospital
- Check glucose if possible

ED Arrival
10 min

3

Immediate general assessment and stabilization
- Assess ABCs, vital signs
- Provide **oxygen** in hypoxemic
- Obtain IV access and perform laboratory assessments
- Check glucose; treat if indicated
- Perform neurologic screening assessment
- Activate stroke team
- Order emergent CT scan or MRI of brain
- Obtain 12-lead ECG

ED Arrival
25 min

4

Immediate neurologic assessment by stroke team or designee
- Review patient history
- Establish time of symptom onset or last know normal
- Perform neurologic examination (NIH Stroke Scale or Canadian Neurological Scale)

Chart Continued on Next Page

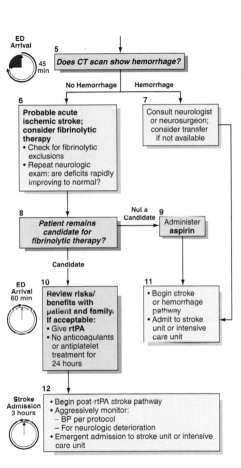

ED Arrival 45 min

5
Does CT scan show hemorrhage?

No Hemorrhage | Hemorrhage

6
Probable acute ischemic stroke; consider fibrinolytic therapy
- Check for fibrinolytic exclusions
- Repeat neurologic exam: are deficits rapidly improving to normal?

7
Consult neurologist or neurosurgeon; consider transfer if not available

8
Patient remains candidate for fibrinolytic therapy?

Not a Candidate

9
Administer aspirin

Candidate

ED Arrival 60 min

10
Review risks/benefits with patient and family. If acceptable:
- Give **rtPA**
- No anticoagulants or antiplatelet treatment for 24 hours

11
- Begin stroke or hemorrhage pathway
- Admit to stroke unit or intensive care unit

Stroke Admission 3 hours

12
- Begin post-rtPA stroke pathway
- Aggressively monitor:
  - BP per protocol
  - For neurologic deterioration
- Emergent admission to stroke unit or intensive care unit

181

REFERENCES

1. Myersburg RJ, Castellanos A: Cardiac arrest and sudden cardiac death. In Zipes DP et al, editors: *Braunwald's heart disease: a textbook of cardiovascular medicine*, ed 7, Philadelphia, 2005, Saunders, pp 865-908.

2. Deleted in 2010 ECC revision.

3. Phalen T, Aehlert B: *The 12-lead ECG in acute coronary syndromes*, St Louis, 2006, Mosby.

4. Deleted in 2010 ECC revision.

5. Deleted in 2010 ECC revision.

6. Deleted in 2010 ECC revision.

7. Deleted in 2010 ECC revision.

8. Vanden Hoek TL, Morrison LJ, Shuster M, et al. Part 12: Cardiac Arrest in Special Situations. 2010 American Heart Association Guidelines for Cardiopulmonary Resuscitation and Emergency Cardiovascular Care. Circulation 2010;122;S829-S861.

9. Vanden Hoek TL, Morrison LJ, Shuster M, et al. Part 12: Cardiac Arrest in Special Situations. 2010 American Heart Association Guidelines for Cardiopulmonary Resuscitation and Emergency Cardiovascular Care. Circulation 2010;122;S829-S861

10. Vanden Hoek TL, Morrison LJ, Shuster M, et al. Part 12: Cardiac Arrest in Special Situations. 2010 American Heart Association Guidelines for Cardiopulmonary Resuscitation and Emergency Cardiovascular Care. Circulation 2010;122;S829-S861.

11. Vanden Hoek TL, Morrison LJ, Shuster M, et al. Part 12: Cardiac Arrest in Special Situations. 2010 American Heart Association Guidelines for Cardiopulmonary Resuscitation and Emergency Cardiovascular Care. Circulation 2010;122;S829-S861

12. Deleted in 2010 ECC revision.

13. Deleted in 2010 ECC revision.

ILLUSTRATION CREDITS

14. Zipes D: *Braunwald's Heart Disease: A Textbook of Cardiovascular Medicine*, ed 7, Philadelphia, 2005, Saunders.

15. Deleted in 2010 ECC revision.

16. Shade B, Rothenberg M, Wertz E, Jones S, and Collins T: *Mosby's EMT-Intermediate Textbook*, ed 2, St. Louis, 2002, Mosby

17. Courtesy LMA North America, Inc.

18. Shade B, Rothenberg M, Wertz E, Jones S, and Collins T: *Mosby's EMT-Intermediate Textbook*, ed 2, St. Louis, 2002, Mosby

19. Urden L, Stacy K, Lough M: *Thelan's Critical Care Nursing: Diagnosis and Management*, ed 5, St. Louis, 2006, Mosby

20. Lounsbury P, Frye S: *Cardiac Rhythm Disorders, A Nursing Approach*, ed 2, St. Louis, 1992, Mosby

21. Thibodeau G, Patton K: *Anatomy & Physiology*, ed 5, St. Louis, 2003, Mosby.

22. Aehlert B: *ECGs Made Easy*, ed 3, St. Louis, 2006, Mosby

23. Crawford MV, Spence MI: *Commonsense Approach to Coronary Care*, rev ed 6, St. Louis, 1994, Mosby.

24. Shade B, Rothenberg M, Wertz E, Jones S, and Collins T: *Mosby's EMT-Intermediate Textbook*, ed 2, St. Louis, 2002, Mosby

25. Goldberger A: *Clinical Electrocardiography: A Simplified Approach*, ed 6, St. Louis, 1999, Mosby

26. Crawford MV, Spence MI: *Commonsense Approach to Coronary Care*, rev ed 6, St. Louis, 1994, Mosby.

27. Surawicz B, Knilans TK: *Chou's electrocardiography in clinical practice: adult and pediatric*, ed 5, Philadelphia, 1996, Saunders.

28. Aehlert B: *ECGs Made Easy*, ed 3, St. Louis, 2006, Mosby

29. Phalen T, Aehlert B: *The 12-Lead ECG in Acute Coronary Syndromes*, ed 2, St. Louis, 2006, Mosby

30. Aehlert B: *ECGs Made Easy Study Cards*, St. Louis, 2004, Mosby

31. Aehlert B: *ECGs Made Easy*, ed 3, St. Louis, 2006, Mosby

32. Shade B, Rothenberg M, Wertz E, Jones S, and Collins T: *Mosby's EMT-Intermediate Textbook*, ed 2, St. Louis, 2002, Mosby

33. Aehlert B: *ECGs Made Easy Study Cards*, St. Louis, 2004, Mosby

34. Aehlert B: *ECGs Made Easy*, ed 3, St. Louis, 2006, Mosby

35. Shade B, Rothenberg M, Wertz E, Jones S, and Collins T: *Mosby's EMT-Intermediate Textbook*, ed 2, St. Louis, 2002, Mosby

36. Aehlert B: *ECGs Made Easy*, ed 3, St. Louis, 2006, Mosby

37. Shade B, Rothenberg M, Wertz E, Jones S, and Collins

T: *Mosby's EMT-Intermediate Textbook*, ed 2, St. Louis, 2002, Mosby

8. Aehlert B: *ECGs Made Easy*, ed 3, St. Louis, 2006, Mosby

9. Grauer K: *A Practical Guide to ECG Interpretation*, ed 2, St. Louis, 1998, Mosby

10. Shade B, Rothenberg M, Wertz E, Jones S, and Collins T: *Mosby's EMT Intermediate Textbook*, ed 2, St. Louis, 2002, Mosby

11. Goldberger A: *Clinical Electrocardiography: A Simplified Approach*, ed 6, St. Louis, 1999, Mosby

12. Cummins R: *ACLS Scenarios: Core Concepts for Case-Based Learning*, St. Louis, 1996, Mosby.

13. Aehlert B: *ECGs Made Easy Study Cards*, St. Louis, 2004, Mosby

14. Aehlert B: *ECGs Made Easy*, ed 3, St. Louis, 2006, Mosby

15. Aehlert B: *ACLS Study Guide*, cd 3, St. Louis, 2007, Mosby.

16. Courtesy Philips Medical Systems

17. Sanders M: *Mosby's Paramedic Textbook*, ed 3, St. Louis, 2005, Mosby

18. Aehlert B: *Mosby's Comprehensive Pediatric Emergency Care*, St. Louis, 2005, Mosby

19. Aehlert B: *ECGs Made Easy*, ed 3, St. Louis, 2006, Mosby

20. Urden L, Stacy K, Lough M: *Thelan's Critical Care Nursing: Diagnosis and Management*, ed 5, St. Louis, 2006, Mosby

21. Butler HA, Caplin M, McCaully E, et al editors: Managing Major Diseases: Cardiac Disorders, vol 2, St. Louis, 1999, Mosby

22. Sanders M: *Mosby's Paramedic Textbook*, ed 3, St. Louis, 2005, Mosby

23. Aehlert B: *ACLS Study Guide*, ed 3, St. Louis, 2007, Mosby.

24. Shade B, Rothenberg M, Wertz E, Jones S, and Collins T: *Mosby's EMT-Intermediate Textbook*, ed 2, St. Louis, 2002, Mosby

25. American Heart Association. *Circulation.* 2010 American Heart Association Guidelines for Cardiopulmonary Resuscitation and Emergency Cardiovascular Care Science. Volume 122, Issue 18, Supplement 3; November 2, 2010.

56. American Heart Association. *Circulation.* 2010 American Heart Association Guidelines for Cardiopulmonary Resuscitation and Emergency Cardiovascular Care Science. Volume 122, Issue 18, Supplement 3; November 2, 2010.

57. American Heart Association. *Circulation.* 2010 American Heart Association Guidelines for Cardiopulmonary Resuscitation and Emergency Cardiovascular Care Science. Volume 122, Issue 18, Supplement 3; November 2, 2010.

58. American Heart Association. *Circulation.* 2010 American Heart Association Guidelines for Cardiopulmonary Resuscitation and Emergency Cardiovascular Care Science. Volume 122, Issue 18, Supplement 3; November 2, 2010.

59. American Heart Association. *Circulation.* 2010 American Heart Association Guidelines for Cardiopulmonary Resuscitation and Emergency Cardiovascular Care Science. Volume 122, Issue 18, Supplement 3; November 2, 2010.

60. American Heart Association. *Circulation.* 2010 American Heart Association Guidelines for Cardiopulmonary Resuscitation and Emergency Cardiovascular Care Science. Volume 122, Issue 18, Supplement 3; November 2, 2010.